Round Table Series 84

Progressing antiseptic development to reduce transmission of antibiotic-resistant pathogens

Edited by

Robert L R Hill

Proceedings of a Round Table discussion held at the Royal College of Surgeons of England in London on 15 December 2005. These discussions reflect the experience and opinions of the panellists and do not necessarily reflect the opinions of the Royal Society of Medicine or the recommendations of Fortis Pharma.

The ROYAL SOCIETY of MEDICINE PRESS Limited

Published by the Royal Society of Medicine Press Ltd
1 Wimpole Street, London W1G 0AE, UK
Tel: +44 (0)20 7290 2921
Fax: +44 (0)20 7290 2929
Email: publishing@rsm.ac.uk
Website: www.rsmpress.co.uk

These proceedings are published by the Royal Society of Medicine Services Ltd with financial support from the sponsor. The contributors are responsible for the scientific content and for the views expressed, which are not necessarily those of the sponsor, of the editor of the series or of the volume, of the Royal Society of Medicine or of the Royal Society of Medicine Press Ltd. Distribution has been in accordance with the wishes of the sponsor but a copy is available to any fellow of the Society at a privileged price.

British Library Cataloguing in Publication Data
A catalogue record for this book is available from the British Library

ISBN 1-85315-634-5
ISSN 0268-3091

Distribution in Europe and Rest of World:
Marston Book Services Ltd
PO Box 269
Abingdon
OXON OX14 4YN, UK
Tel: +44 (0)1235 465 500
Fax: +44 (0)1235 465 555
Email: direct.order@marston.co.uk

Distribution in Australia and New Zealand:
Elsevier Australia
30–52 Smidmore Street
Marrickville NSW 2204
Australia
Tel: + 61 2 9517 8999
Fax: + 61 2 9517 2249
Email: service@elsevier.com.au

Distribution in the USA and Canada:
Royal Society of Medicine Press Ltd
c/o BookMasters, Inc
30 Amberwood Parkway
Ashland, Ohio 44805, USA
Tel: +1 800 247 6553 / +1 800 266 5564
E-mail: order@bookmasters.com

Phototypeset by Phoenix Photosetting, Chatham, Kent

Printed by Alden Press, Oxford

Contents

Contributors and participants

Zainab Al-Doori
Scottish MRSA Reference Laboratory, Stobhill Hospital, Glasgow, UK

Graham Ayliffe
Emeritus Professor of Medical Microbiology, University of Birmingham; formerly Director, Hospital Infection Research Laboratory, City Hospital, Birmingham, UK

Richard A Bojar
Skin Research Centre, Institute of Molecular and Cellular Biology, Faculty of Biological Sciences, University of Leeds, Leeds, UK

Martina Cummins
School of Nursing and Midwifery, City University, London, UK

Dinah Gould
School of Nursing and Midwifery, City University, London, UK

Robert LR Hill
Senior Lecturer, Guy's, King's and St Thomas' School of Medicine; currently Head, Antibiotic Resistance Evaluation, Centre for Infections, Colindale, London, UK

Keith T Holland
Skin Research Centre, Institute of Molecular and Cellular Biology, Faculty of Biological Sciences, University of Leeds, Leeds, UK

Angela M Kearns
Head, Staphylococcal Reference Unit, Centre for Infections, Colindale, London, UK

Donald Morrison
Scottish MRSA Reference Laboratory, Stobhill Hospital, Glasgow, UK

Judith Tanner
Lead for Nursing Research, Derby Hospitals NHS Foundations Trust

Introduction

Graham Ayliffe

At the beginning of the 20th century, aseptic surgical methods gradually replaced the antiseptic technique of Lister in the prevention of wound infection, but antiseptics were still required for disinfection of hands and operation sites. Scrubbing with soap and water, followed by an alcohol rinse, was generally used for presurgical hand preparation, and alcoholic iodine or a quaternary ammonium compound was used for disinfection of the operation site. Despite the work of Semmelweiss on prevention of puerperal fever in the mid-19th century, the importance of hand disinfection to prevent cross-infection in wards received little attention until the outbreaks of penicillin-resistant *Staphylococcus aureus* infections in the 1950s.

At this time, an antistaphylococcal agent, hexachlorophane, was introduced for staff handwashing, for postoperative bathing of patients and as a powder for application to babies' umbilical sites. It was also useful for adding to bathwater to prevent infection of open wounds and for the treatment of staphylococcal skin carriers. Although it had a good residual effect, its use was mainly discontinued (apart from the powder) in the early 1970s due to neurotoxicity in neonates when bathed with the detergent preparation.

Hexachlorophane was mainly replaced by chlorhexidine and povidone-iodine, and to a lesser extent by triclosan for skin disinfection, both in wards and in operating theatres. These agents are relatively non-toxic and non-allergenic and have been in continual use since then. More recently, 70% ethanol and 60% isopropanol, with or without another added antiseptic agent, were introduced for hand disinfection in wards as well as in theatres. As yet there appears to be no evidence of emergence of clinically relevant resistance of *S. aureus* to these agents and no important alternative new products have emerged over the past 50 years.

The possible advantages and disadvantages of alcohols over antiseptic detergents for hand disinfection continue to be discussed. Continental Europeans have long favoured alcohols, and these are now being more widely used in the UK and the USA.

The prevention of the spread of epidemic methicillin-resistant *S. aureus* (MRSA) remains a problem. The reason why cross-infection is so difficult to control when compared with previous outbreaks of MRSA and other antibiotic-resistant strains remains uncertain, particularly when similar apparently effective methods of control are still available. The cause of the worldwide epidemic of MRSA appears to be multifactorial – e.g. differences in hospital organization, patient and staff movements between wards, mixtures of differing types of patient in the same wards, older populations of patients, more invasive procedures, increase in carriers in the community and their readmission to hospitals, failure of isolation of infected patients, and failure of implementation of hand disinfection by staff after contact with infected patients. The hospital environment probably plays a minor role in the spread of MRSA. However, it is also possible that the properties of epidemic strains have changed. There could be an undetected transmissibility factor, longer survival in the environment may be of relevance, or strains with undetected resistance to existing antiseptics, in addition to antibiotics, could have recently emerged.

Less attention is probably being paid to the detection and treatment of carriers and dispersers and to the airborne spread of contaminated skin scales. *S. aureus* can spread by multiple routes. Hands may be the most important mode of spread, but there are alternative routes, especially if one is blocked. Indeed, hands cannot always be washed/disinfected after every patient contact due to lack of time for staff working in busy units. Priorities need to be established in this 'grey' area, instead of continuing the failure of attempts to achieve full implementation following every patient contact.

In the 1960s, Lowbury and Lilly described methods for hygienic hand washing/disinfection (i.e. removal or killing of transients) and surgical hand washing/disinfection (i.e. removal and/or killing of residents and transients) using laboratory volunteers. However, in recent years, European experts have described rather similar tests that are now approved by the European Union as EN Standards. These tests have problems in clinical interpretation. For example, *Escherichia coli* is used as the test organism for hygienic disinfection, but it dies rapidly on drying and the application time in the test is 1 minute, compared with 15–20 seconds in practice. Alcohols are significantly more effective than antiseptic detergents in these laboratory tests with volunteers. They show a 3–4 log reduction, whereas antiseptic detergents show a 2–3 log reduction, and soap and water a 2 log reduction. However, does statistical significance correspond to clinical significance and are these differences sufficient to influence prevention of cross-infection? Alcohols are inappropriate for open wounds and are not effective against bacterial spores and some viruses. Some detergent-based agents such as chlorhexidine show a good residual effect compared with alcoholic preparations. Is this of clinical relevance?

Highly resistant Gram-negative bacilli are causing more infections. *Clostridium difficile* is emerging as a significant pathogen. Can we use antiseptics to influence their spread?

Many of these and other problems are discussed in this publication.

- The recently described community-associated MRSA (CA-MRSA) is discussed by Angela Kearns. These strains are particularly virulent and in this respect resemble the original phage type 80/81 strains.
- Dinah Gould reviews her work on methods of promoting hygienic hand disinfection and improving compliance as well as other aspects of control of infection.
- Judith Tanner discusses the preliminary findings of the Cochrane review of surgical hand disinfection and identifies areas of future research.
- Zainab Al-Doori and Donald Morrison describe a new ex-vivo skin method for testing biocides and its application in determining resistance of MRSA to antiseptics.
- Keith Holland and Richard Bojar evaluate existing methods of testing antiseptics and also describe a new technique, the skin equivalent method, which should give realistic results on microbiological testing of biocides and resistance of MRSA to antiseptics. They also discuss the determination of skin irritancy.
- Robert Hill describes a human model for analysing the potential role of the antiseptic half-life of antiseptics on the skin in the prevention of infection in the presence of non-compliant hand hygiene. He also describes the use of pig skin for testing antibiotic-resistant strains.
- Finally, Martina Cummins compares EMRSA at the London Hospital in the 1980s with today. She shows the effectiveness of enhanced screening, treatment of carriers and the use of an isolation ward in maintaining a low level of EMRSA over the years.

True community MRSA: Current status and opportunities for infection control

Angela M Kearns

Over the last two decades, 17 strains of epidemic methicillin-resistant *Staphylococcus aureus* (MRSA) have been identified in UK healthcare settings. More recently, different MRSA strains have evolved in the community. These community-associated MRSA (CA-MRSA) have been recovered from previously healthy individuals without the classical risk factors for MRSA infection, such as recent hospitalization, nursing home residence or prior antimicrobial therapy.

CA-MRSA most commonly cause skin and soft tissue infection (particularly boils and abscesses), but necrotizing pneumonia associated with a high fatality rate has also been reported. The increasing frequency of CA-MRSA causing sporadic disease in the community, and outbreaks of infection among prison inmates, among men who have sex with men and among athletic teams, suggest that a new pattern of staphylococcal disease is emerging, presenting a new public health challenge.

Continued vigilance for CA-MRSA is essential to increase our understanding of the epidemiology and risk factors, and to help inform infection control and patient management strategies.

Background

MRSA is a major cause of healthcare-associated infection worldwide. Following the first reports of UK epidemic MRSA (EMRSA) in the early 1980s, 17 strains (EMRSA-1 to -17) have been identified in UK healthcare settings.[1,2] Currently, two major clones predominate in hospitals in the UK: EMRSA-15 and -16.[3]

Although most human infections are thought to be nosocomial, community-acquired MRSA infections are being reported increasingly. MRSA occurring in the community was observed in 1980 following an outbreak among injecting drug users in Detroit.[4] Subsequently, cases of community-associated MRSA (CA-MRSA), as distinct from healthcare-associated MRSA (HA-MRSA), have been reported in the UK and worldwide, causing international concern.[5–17] In contrast to HA-MRSA, these organisms have been identified in individuals without established risk factors for MRSA infection, such as residence in long-term care facilities, recent hospitalization, surgery or injecting drug use,[8,18,19] suggesting that a new pattern of disease may be emerging.

Various studies have sought to establish the nasal carriage rate of MRSA in the community. Figures vary widely according to the different locations and populations surveyed. Based on estimates from meta-analyses, the nasal colonization rate for MRSA is 1.3% among individuals in the community.[20] Excluding individuals with HA-MRSA risk factors (in an attempt to give more accurate figures for true CA-MRSA) yields estimates that are considerably lower ($\leqslant$0.024%).[20]

CA-MRSA

There is much confusion regarding the origin of MRSA in the community. Patients with HA-MRSA may be discharged from hospital resulting in 'overspill' of these organisms into the community setting.[21] Consequently, prior healthcare exposure may lead to misidentification of HA-MRSA occurring in the community as CA-MRSA. Various authors have acknowledged the difficulties in establishing whether isolates are genuine HA-MRSA or CA-MRSA, even when healthcare-associated risk factors are rigorously assessed,[10,19,22] leading to an overestimate of the prevalence of true CA-MRSA.[10,19,20] Set against this background, it is becoming increasingly apparent that it is not possible to define CA-MRSA solely on the basis of demographic and epidemiological information.

There is now clear genetic-based evidence that *bona fide* CA-MRSA strains are distinct from HA-MRSA.[8,13,22] Therefore, to accurately identify isolates of community origin as CA-MRSA and differentiate them reliably from HA-MRSA, microbiological analyses are essential.[8,11,23]

Characteristics of CA-MRSA

True CA-MRSA possess a number of features that differentiate them from HA-MRSA: susceptibility to most antimicrobials other than β-lactams, DNA fingerprinting profiles distinct from those of HA-MRSA,[8,11,24] carriage of staphylococcal chromosome cassette *mec* (SCC*mec*) type IV or V (see below) and presence of Panton-Valentine leukocidin genes in some lineages (see below).

Staphylococcal cassette chromosome *mec* (SCC*mec*)

Methicillin resistance is encoded by the *mecA* gene, which is located on a mobile genetic element known as staphylococcal cassette chromosome *mec* (SCC*mec*). Five different SCC*mec* elements (I to V) have been characterized that vary in size, composition and organization. SCC*mec* types IV and V have been associated with CA-MRSA.[24,25] In addition, several subtypes of SCC*mec* type IV have been identified on the basis of DNA sequence polymorphism within this element.[22,26] Polymerase chain reaction-based strategies have been designed to assist with the identification of CA-MRSA, and to characterize the structural type of SCC*mec* found in these strains.[24,25] SCC*mec* typing,[24–26] together with multilocus sequence typing (MLST),[27] provide a standardized nomenclature for the characterization and comparison of these strains internationally.

Panton-Valentine leukocidin

In 1932, Panton and Valentine described the activity of a leukocidin, now known as Panton-Valentine leukocidin (PVL), in a strain of *S. aureus* from a case of chronic furunculosis.[28] It is now known that PVL is encoded by two cotranscribed genes (*lukS-PV* and *lukF-PV*) found on several temperate bacteriophages.[29] Few strains appear to be susceptible to infection with PVL-converting phages,[29] which probably accounts for the relatively low frequency (1.6–10%) of clinical isolates of *S. aureus* found to harbour the PVL genes.[12,30] PVL induces pore formation in leukoctyes, triggering the release of interleukins and other inflammatory mediators, leading to tissue necrosis and abscess formation.[22,31] This toxin is now regarded as a marker of virulence in CA-MRSA, although it is not believed to be the sole pathogenic determinant.[22]

Data show that CA-MRSA exhibit considerable genetic heterogeneity. Multiple independent clonal lineages of CA-MRSA have been reported in the UK and worldwide, suggesting they have arisen from diverse genetic backgrounds rather than from the worldwide spread of a single clone.[8,11,22,23] Given their distinct genetic backgrounds, CA-MRSA are believed to have evolved independently of HA-MRSA.[23] The work of Robinson *et al*[32] supports this hypothesis. Backed by detailed interstrain comparative data, the authors showed that one of the CA-MRSA clones found in the Southern Pacific and elsewhere[8,11,23] is derived from the so-called phage type 80/81 methicillin-sensitive *S. aureus* (MSSA) strains prevalent in the 1950s and 1960s, which caused a pandemic of community-acquired severe skin and soft tissue infections (SSTIs), pneumonias and septicaemias in children and young adults. These observations suggest that CA-MRSA may have evolved from successful MSSA found in the community following acquisition of methicillin resistance.[32]

Changing pattern of disease

CA-MRSA have been associated with considerable morbidity and mortality worldwide. Epidemiological data show that they are strongly associated with SSTIs, most commonly presenting as primary, often necrotic, cutaneous lesions (e.g. boils, abscesses and furuncles), which may require surgical incision and drainage.[6–8,14,18,33,34] Although predominantly responsible for sporadic disease in previously healthy individuals in the community, outbreaks of SSTIs due to CA-MRSA have been reported among prison inmates, men who have sex with men, close-contact sporting groups (e.g. football and rugby), military recruits, injecting drug users, schoolchildren and newborn babies.[4,6,7,31] Of further concern are reports of CA-MRSA associated with life-threatening, invasive disease. In particular, fatal cases of severe sepsis, community-acquired necrotizing pneumonia and purpura fulminans due to CA-MRSA have been described in previously healthy paediatric patients and young adults without known hospital contact.[5,35,36] Collectively, reports of CA-MRSA causing infection outside traditional healthcare settings herald a change in the pathogenesis and epidemiology of MRSA worldwide.

CA-MRSA in England and Wales

CA-MRSA were reported as early as 1996 in the UK, causing abscesses in rugby players from the South Pacific.[37] Subsequently, there have been a number of cases of CA-MRSA infection occurring in England and Wales.[9,12,16,17]

Using detailed microbiological analyses[12] the Staphylococcus Reference Unit (Centre for Infections, Health Protection Agency, London) has identified in excess of 300 isolates of CA-MRSA among cultures referred from throughout England and Wales over a 2-year period (2004–2005). These figures are likely to reflect an underestimate of the prevalence of CA-MRSA, since not all patients presenting with an infection will have a sample sent to the laboratory for microbiological testing; factors such as local policies, severity of infection, failure to respond to therapy and so on are likely to influence sample referral.

The microbiological data show that the isolates comprise seven distinct genetic lineages (Table 1). Five of the clones have been found to encode the PVL genes (ST8-MRSA-SCC*mec*IVa, ST22-MRSA-SCC*mec*IVA, ST30-MRSA-SCC*mec*IVc, ST80-MRSA-SCC*mec*IVc and ST88-MRSA-SCC*mec*IVa). Most of these clonal lineages have been reported to occur in other areas, such as the USA, Southern Pacific and Europe.[8,9,11,23,33,34,38] The two remaining clones have proved to be PVL-naive (ST1-MRSA-SCC*mec*IVa and ST5-MRSA-SCC*mec*IVa), and have been reported in countries such as Australia and Portugal.[8,23,39] From the clinical data available, the majority of CA-MRSA isolates (about 60%) have been associated with SSTIs (predominantly abscesses, boils and skin lesions). In some instances, infections appear to have been imported, while others have been acquired domestically. Most of the cases have been distributed throughout England and Wales and appear to be unrelated epidemiologically.

In general, each of the seven clones exhibits a characteristic antibiogram (Table 1). In addition to β-lactam resistance, the strains display resistance to up to two other antimicrobial agents – specifically fusidic acid, erythromycin, gentamicin, tetracycline and/or (rarely) ciprofloxacin. A useful phenotypic marker for recognizing putative CA-MRSA in the clinical diagnostic laboratory, therefore, is susceptibility to ciprofloxacin – a feature uncommon among UK HA-MRSA strains. However, for definitive microbiological confirmation of CA-MRSA, molecular strain characterization data remain essential.

CA-MRSA in healthcare settings

While HA-MRSA remains a serious threat to hospitalized patients, there have been reports from several countries of CA-MRSA infiltrating the healthcare environment with onward nosocomial transmission.[40–42] The extent to which CA-MRSA strains are displacing HA-MRSA or adding to the overall burden of MRSA as causes of infection in hospitals is currently unknown, but these are worrying developments and present a new challenge for public health personnel. Moreover, exposure to antimicrobial use in the healthcare environment has the potential to select for multidrug-resistant CA-MRSA, and these have already been reported in some countries.[15,23]

Patient management and infection control issues

Early diagnosis and improvements in CA-MRSA case ascertainment are required from a clinical and therapeutic perspective. Systematic studies are called for – not only to give accurate estimates of the prevalence of CA-MRSA in community and healthcare settings in the UK, but also to monitor for associated risk factors and the emergence of more virulent and/or multiresistant clones. Such studies would provide valuable information to help underpin therapeutic and patient management strategies. In particular, susceptibility testing data would help establish whether the empirical use of β-lactams for community-associated *S. aureus* infections remains prudent.

CA-MRSA as a cause of outbreaks and sporadic disease raises important questions relating to the need for infection control strategies targeted towards these organisms nationally and internationally. Interim guidelines for the management of CA-MRSA have been proposed (e.g. http://www.metrokc.gov/health/providers/epidemiology/MRSA-guidelines.pdf). In the UK, guidelines for the control of HA-

TABLE 1 Characteristics of CA-MRSA clones in England and Wales

	CA-MRSA characteristics						
Multilocus sequence type	ST1	ST5	ST8	ST22	ST30	ST80	ST88
SCC*mec* type[a]	IVa	IVa	IVa	IVA	IVc	IVc	IVa
Toxin gene profile[b]	Enterotoxins A and H	Enterotoxins D, G, I and J	PVL	PVL; enterotoxins G and I	PVL, enterotoxins G and I	PVL, enterotoxin H;[c] exfoliative toxin D	PVL
Antimicrobial susceptibility[d]							
β-lactams	R	R	R	R	R	R	R
Ciprofloxacin	S	S	V	S	S	S	S
Fusidic acid	R	S	S	S	S	R	S
Tetracycline	S	R	S	S	R	V	R
Erythromycin	V	S	V	S	R	S	S
Gentamicin	S	S	S	R	S	S	S

[a] After the nomenclature of Oliveira *et al*[25] and Huletsky *et al*[26].

[b] 14 toxin genes screened for[12] (PVL; enterotoxins A–E and G–J; toxic shock syndrome toxin 1; exfoliative toxins A, B and D).

[c] Variable trait.

[d] R, resistant; S, susceptible; V, variable

MRSA in hospitals and the community have been published.[1,21] However, it is not yet clear whether infection control programmes developed for tackling threats posed by healthcare-associated pathogens are appropriate or need to be reformulated to take account of the emergence of CA-MRSA in community and healthcare environments. Interestingly, countries with a low prevalence of HA-MRSA, such as Denmark, have recently reported the infiltration of CA-MRSA, suggesting that well-established infection control measures designed for HA-MRSA need to be reviewed to contain the spread of CA-MRSA.[34]

In designing prevention and infection control measures for CA-MRSA, consideration needs to be given to identifiable risk factors. To date, outbreaks have been described particularly where individuals are in close contact, where there is risk of skin trauma and where personal items are likely to be shared.[6,7,37,38,40] Extrapolating from guidelines for the control of HA-MRSA in hospital and community settings, simple interventions such as handwashing, attention to good standards of hygiene, occluding skin lesions (cuts, wounds, etc.) with an impermeable dressing and avoidance of sharing personal items (e.g. towels and razors) to limit CA-MRSA transmission are advisable.[1,21]

The attempted eradication of MRSA carriage to reduce the burden of HA- and CA-MRSA is a controversial issue.[1,22] Not only can decolonization be difficult to achieve, but the possible emergence of antimicrobial resistance is an additional concern.[1,21,22,43] The majority of CA-MRSA infections in England and Wales are sporadic in nature, and it is not currently clear whether screening of close contacts should be advocated and, where positive, decolonization attempted. In a community-based cluster of CA-MRSA in Denmark, efforts were made to decolonize individuals using a combination of daily showers with chlorhexidine detergent in addition to nasal mupirocin, together with household hygienic measures.[43] The findings show that eradication of CA-MRSA can be as challenging as the attempted eradication of HA-MRSA.[1,38,43] Additional evidence-based data are required, but, in view of the morbidity and mortality associated with CA-MRSA, screening and decolonization of individuals and their close contacts would seem prudent, particularly where infections are recurrent or life-threatening, or where there are clusters of disease.[22,43]

In conclusion, CA-MRSA is becoming an increasing public health problem worldwide. This is a worrying trend, and healthcare personnel need to be cognisant of these changes in the epidemiology of MRSA. Moreover, systematic studies are required not only to increase our understanding of the epidemiology, pathogenicity, antimicrobial susceptibility, and prevalence of CA-MRSA, but also to identify risk factors and effective prevention and control strategies to limit their spread.

References

1. Ayliffe GAJ, Buckles A, Casewell MW et al. on behalf of the working party of the British Society of Antimicrobial Chemotherapy, the Hospital Infection Society and the Infection Control Nurses Association. Revised guidelines for the control of methicillin-resistant *Staphylococcus aureus* infection in hospitals. *J Hosp Infect* 1998;**39**:253–90.

2. Aucken HM, Ganner M, Murchan S, Cookson BD, Johnson AP. A new strain of epidemic methicillin-resistant *Staphylococcus aureus* (EMRSA-17) resistant to multiple antibiotics. *J Antimicrob Chemother* 2002;**50**:171–5.

3. Johnson AP, Aucken HM, Vavendish S et al, and the UK EARSS participants. Dominance of EMRSA-15 and -16 among MRSA causing nosocomial bacteraemia in the UK: analysis of isolates from the European Antimicrobial Resistance Surveillance System (EARSS). *J Antimicrob Chemother* 2001;**48**:143–4.

4. Saravolatz LD, Markowitz N, Arking L, Pohlod D, Fisher E. Methicillin resistant *Staphylococcus aureus*: epidemiologic observations during a community-acquired outbreak. *Ann Intern Med* 1982;**96**:11–16.

5. Centers for Disease Control and Prevention. Four paediatric deaths from community-acquired methicillin-resistant *Staphylococcus aureus* – Minnesota and North Dakota, 1997–1999. *Morb Mortal Wkly Rep* 1999;**48**:707–10.

6. Centers for Disease Control and Prevention. Methicillin-resistant *Staphylococcus aureus* infections among competitive sports participants – Colorado, Indiana, Pennsylvania, and Los Angeles County, 2000–2003. *Morb Mortal Wkly Rep* 2003;**52**:793–95.

7. Centers for Disease Control and Prevention. Outbreaks of community-associated methicillin-resistant *Staphylococcus aureus* skin infections – Los Angeles County, California, 2002–2003. *Morb Mortal Wkly Rep* 2003;**52**:88.

8. Vandenesch F, Naimi T, Enright MC et al. Community-acquired methicillin-resistant *Staphylococcus aureus* carrying Panton-Valentine leukocidin genes: worldwide emergence. *Emerg Infect Dis* 2003;**9**:978–84.

9. Kearns AM, Rathmann IR, Holmes A, Pitt TL, Cookson BD. An unusual clone of MRSA causing infection in injecting drug users. *J Infect* 2004;**49**:49–50.

10. Harbarth S, Francois P, Schrenzel J et al. Community-associated methicillin-resistant *Staphylococcus aureus*, Switzerland. *Emerg Infect Dis* 2005;**11**:962–5.

11. Health Protection Agency. Community MRSA in England and Wales: definition through strain characterisation. *CDR Weekly* 2005;**15**:3–4.

12. Holmes A, Ganner M, McGuane S, Pitt TL, Cookson BD, Kearns AM. *Staphylococcus aureus* carrying Panton-Valentine leukocidin genes (PVL) in England and Wales: frequency, characterisation and association with clinical disease. *J Clin Microbiol* 2005;**43**:2384–90.

13. Ma XX, Galiana A, Pedreira W et al. Community-acquired methicillin-resistant *Staphylococcus aureus*, Uruguay. *Emerg Infect Dis* 2005;**11**:973–6.

14. Moran GJ, Amii RN, Abrahamian FM, Talan DA. Methicillin-resistant *Staphylococcus aureus* in community-acquired skin infections. *Emerg Infect Dis* 2005;**11**:928–30.

15. Mulvey MR, MacDougall L, Cholin B, Horsman G, Fidyk M, Woods S, and the Saskatchewan CA-MRSA Study Group. Community-associated methicillin-resistant *Staphylococcus aureus*, Canada. *Emerg Infect Dis* 2005;**11**:844–50.

16. Reichert B, Birrell G, Bignardi G. Severe non-pneumonic necrotising infections in children caused by Panton-Valentine leukocidin producing *Staphylococcus aureus*. *J Infect* 2005; **50**: 438–42.

17. Jeyaratnam D, Reid C, Kearns AM, Klein JL. Community-associated MRSA: an alert to paediatricians. *Arch Dis Child* (in press).

18. Naimi TS, LeDell KH, Boxrud DJ et al. Epidemiology and clonality of community-associated methicillin-resistant *Staphylococcus aureus* in Minnesota, 1996–1998. *Clin Infect Dis* 2001;**33**:990–6.

19. Folden DV, Machayya JA, Sahmoun AE et al. Estimating the proportion of community-associated methicillin-resistant *Staphylococcus aureus*: two definitions used in the USA yield dramatically different estimates. *J Hosp Infect* 2005;**60**:329–32.

20. Salgado CD, Farr BM, Calfee DP. Community-acquired methicillin-resistant *Staphylococcus aureus*: a meta-analysis of prevalence and risk factors. *Clin Infect Dis* 2003;**36**:131–9.

21. Report of a combined working party for the British Society for Antimicrobial Chemotherapy and the Hospital Infection Society. Guidelines on the control of methicillin-resistant *Staphylococcus aureus* in the community. *J Hosp Infect* 1995;**31**:1–12.

22. Zetola N, Francis JS, Nuermberger EL, Bishai WR. Community-acquired methicillin-resistant *Staphylococcus aureus*: an emerging threat. *Lancet Infect Dis 2005*;**5**:275–86.

23. Coombs GW, Pearson JC, O'Brien FG, Murray RJ, Grubb WB, Christiansen KJ. Methicillin-resistant *Staphylococcus aureus* clones, Western Australia. *Emerg Infect Dis* 2006;**12**:241–7.

24. Ito T, Ma XX, Takeuchi F, Okuma K, Ciu L, Hiramatsu K. Novel type V staphylococcal cassette chromosome *mec* driven by a novel cassette chromosome recombinase *ccrC*. *J Clin Microbiol* 2004;**48**:2637–51.

25. Oliveira DC, de Lencastre H. Multiplex PCR strategy for rapid identification of structural types and variants of the *mec* element in methicillin-resistant *Staphylococcus aureus*. *Antimicrob Agents Chemother* 2002;**46**:2155–61.

26. Huletsky A, Giroux R, Rossbach V et al. New real-time PCR assay for rapid detection of methicillin-resistant *Staphylococcus aureus* directly from specimens containing a mixture of staphylococci. *J Clin Microbiol* 2004;**42:**1875–84.

27. Enright MC, Day NP, Davies CE, Peacock SJ, Spratt BG. Multilocus sequence typing for characterization of methicillin-resistant and methicillin-susceptible clones of *Staphylococcus aureus*. *J Clin Microbiol* 2000;**38**:1008–15.

28. Panton PN, Valentine FCO. Staphylococcal toxin. *Lancet* 1932;**222(i)**:506–8.

29. Narita S, Kaneko J, Chiba J et al. Phage conversion of Panton-Valentine leukocidin in *Staphylococcus aureus*: molecular analysis of a PVL-converting phage, ϕSLT. *Gene* 2001;**268**:195–206.

30. Prévost G, Couppie P, Prévost P et al. Epidemiological data on *Staphylococcus aureus* strains producing syngohymenotropic toxins. *J Med Microbiol* 1995**42**:237–45.

31. Francis JS, Doherty MC, Lopatin U et al. Severe community-onset pneumonia in healthy adults caused by methicillin-resistant *Staphylococcus aureus* carrying the Panton-Valentine leukocidin genes. *Clin Infect Dis* 2005;**40**:100–7.

32. Robinson DA, Kearns AM, Holmes A et al. Re-emergence of early pandemic *Staphylococcus aureus* as a community-acquired methicillin-resistant clone. *Lancet* 2005:**365**;1256–8.

33. Witte W, Braulke C, Cuny C et al. Emergence of methicillin-resistant *Staphylococcus aureus* with Panton-Valentine leukocidin genes in central Europe. *Eur J Clin Microbiol Infect Dis* 2005;**24**:1–5.

34. Faria NA, Oliviera DC, Westh H et al. Epidemiology of emerging methicillin-resistant *Staphylococcus aureus* (MRSA) in Denmark: a nationwide study in a country with low prevalence of MRSA infection. *J Clin Microbiol* 2005;**43**:1836–42.

35. Gillet Y, Issartel B, Vanhems P et al. Association between *Staphylococcus aureus* strains carrying gene for Panton-Valentine leukocidin and highly lethal necrotising pneumonia in young immunocompetent patients. *Lancet* 2002;**359**:753–9.

36. Kravitz GR, Dries DJ, Peterson ML, Schlievert PM. Purpura fulminans due to *Staphylococcus aureus*. *Clin Infect Dis* 2005;**40**:941–7.

37. Stacey AR, Endersby KE, Chan PC, Marples RR. An outbreak of methicillin-resistant *Staphylococcus aureus* infection in a rugby football team. *Br J Sports Med* 1998;**32**:153–4.

38. Urth T, Juul G, Skov R, Schønheyder HC. Spread of a methicillin-resistant *Staphylococcus aureus* ST80-IV clone in a Danish community. *Infect Control Hosp Epidemiol* 2005;**26**:144–9.

39. Sá-leão R, Santos Sanches I, Dias D, Peres I, Barros RM, de Lencastre H. Detection of an archaic clone of *Staphylococcus aureus* with low level resistance to methicillin in a pediatric hospital in Portugal and in international samples: relics of a formerly widely disseminated strain? *J Clin Microbiol* 1999;**37**:1913–20.

40. Saiman L, O'Keefe M, Graham PL III et al. Hospital transmission of community-acquired methicillin-resistant *Staphylococcus aureus* among postpartum women. *Clin Infect Dis* 2003;**37**:1313–19.

41. Kourbatova EV, Halvosa JS, King MD, Ray SM, White N, Blumberg HM. Emergence of community-associated methicillin-resistant *Staphylococcus aureus* USA 300 clone as a cause of health care-associated infections among patients with prosthetic joint infections. *Am J Infect Control* 2005;**33**:385–91.

42. Klevens RM, Edwards JR, Tenover FC, McDonald LC, Horan T, Gaynes R and the National Nosocomial Infections Surveillance System. Changes in the epidemiology of methicillin-resistant *Staphylococcus aureus* in intensive care units in US hospitals, 1992–2003. *Clin Infect Dis* 2006;**42**:389–91.

43. Kniehl E, Becker A, Forster DH. Bed, bath and beyond: pitfalls in prompt eradication of methicillin-resistant *Staphylococcus aureus* carrier status in healthcare workers. *J Hosp Infect* 2005;**59**:180–7.

Discussion

ROBERT HILL: The epidemiology of MRSA is clearly changing internationally, and it is important to realize this. What do you feel is the value of discriminating true community MRSA from hospital MRSA?

ANGELA KEARNS: Well, the management of true community MRSA will be different, due to the difference in virulence. We need to know if a strain is a true community strain, and, if so, where has it come from.

KEITH HOLLAND: I am not totally convinced that Panton-Valentine leukocidin (PVL) is the only virulence marker. This organism is so complex in its regulation of virulence that other, as yet undiscovered factors, may discriminate a community from a hospital strain. Discovering these may usefully guide management strategies. I do agree that action needs to be taken once a family has been screened and cases of CA-MRSA identified – academic interest is not going to be good enough for the family involved.

ANGELA KEARNS: One of the interesting aspects emerging from our work is that PVL positivity is not necessarily associated with nasal carriage. Carriage may be via other sites such as the armpit or groin. Healthcare guidelines for hospital strains that recommend nasal swabbing may not be appropriate for CA-MRSA.

KEITH HOLLAND: So there may be different adhesion factors for CA-MRSA compared with HA-MRSA, giving CA-MRSA an advantage in the locations that you mentioned?

ANGELA KEARNS: Absolutely – the whole picture is much more complex than I have been able to present; for example, two of the most common CA-MRSA strains are PVL-negative, so I agree that there may be virulence cofactors that have not yet been identified.

GRAHAM AYLIFFE: The virulent strains that you describe resemble the original phage type 80/81 strains (in the 1940s and 1950s). Phage type 80 was particularly virulent, causing sepsis in neonatal units, breast abscesses in mothers, and furunculosis and septic fingers in staff – who were often nasal carriers. Chlorhexidine baths proved remarkably effective in preventing spread.

DONALD MORRISION: Current CA-MRSA outbreaks can be challenging to control. In one recent example, CA-MRSA was identified in a Glaswegian family. It took a year to decolonize them – the process involved extensive decolonization of their domestic environment, including changing their furniture.

KEITH HOLLAND: Could small colony variants also be playing a role? If CA-MRSA strains are persisting, perhaps they are hiding in cells, occasionally becoming aggressive.

ANGELA KEARNS: There has to have been a reservoir somewhere for these persistent relapsing infections that can take a very long time to clear.

KEITH HOLLAND: I would not be surprised to find that these organisms are getting into keratinocytes, but I have no data to support such a hypothesis.

ROBERT HILL: True CA-MRSA is extremely interesting – it differs from the HA-MRSA we are used to. CA-MRSA produces much more serious problems and poses a challenge for infection control in the community.

Hand washing as a basis for infection control

Dinah Gould

Hygienic hand disinfection is at the forefront of current strategies to control infection. Alcohol-based products are promoted as the most effective. However, despite excellent bactericidal properties, they do not destroy spores and some important viruses. Despite rapid action, their effectiveness is short-lived and depends on high levels of health worker compliance, with care taken to ensure that all hand surfaces receive contact before evaporation. In practice, this is difficult to achieve, especially at busy times when greatest reliance is placed on alcohol-based products. There is a lack of practical evidence-based guidance concerning the correct use of these products to ensure safe practice, and an assumption that models of infection control which work in other countries will translate equally well into the United Kingdom (UK) National Health Service (NHS).

Introduction

Antiseptics used for hygienic hand decontamination (HHD) are at the forefront of current strategies to reduce healthcare-associated infection (HCAI) in the UK.[1,2] In recent years, alcohol-based products have gained increasing popularity and their use is now being heavily promoted as part of the CleanYourHandsCampaign (CYHC) introduced throughout England and Wales in the spring of 2005.[3] Nevertheless, infections caused by multiply-resistant pathogens continue to be reported and remain a major cause of concern to health professionals and the public.[4] This has prompted the following questions:

- Are alcohol-based products the best choice for routine HHD?
- How effective are alcohol-based products when used routinely by practitioners?
- Is there enough guidance about how alcohol-based products should be used to achieve safe practice?
- Is HHD still the single most important infection control procedure in the NHS today?
- What factors in addition to poor compliance with HHD may be contributing to the relatively high rates of HCAI recorded in the UK compared with continental Europe, where alcohol-based products are the mainstay of infection control?

Are alcohol-based products the best choice for routine hygienic hand disinfection?

Hand washing has long been considered the single most effective and cost-effective way of controlling cross-infection.[5–7] A number of products are available, including non-medicated soaps, aqueous antiseptic solutions and alcohol-based products.

Soaps

These have a detergent effect. They remove transient microorganisms physically, but have no effect on the resident microbial population. Unlike antiseptics, they are not bactericidal and cannot inhibit bacterial growth, which limits their effectiveness.[8] Nevertheless, liquid soap is still perfectly adequate when performing routine hand washing in low-risk situations, providing it is dispensed from a sealed cartridge preventing contamination. Today, health workers are required to perform an increasing number of invasive procedures that require gloves. Soap is not the best choice on these occasions, because conditions beneath the glove encourage bacteria to be leached out of the subungual spaces, increasing the number that may contribute to cross-infection.[9] A disinfectant would be better, especially a long-acting one.

Aqueous antiseptic products

These bring about a greater reduction in the number of transient and resident micro-organisms than soap, either by killing or by inhibiting their growth.[8] Some antiseptics have a detergent effect or are marketed in a formulation that includes a detergent, and these are suitable for use on hands that are visibly soiled. The most commonly used aqueous antiseptic products in the UK employ Chlorhexidine gluconate, povidone-iodine or triclosan as the active ingredient.

Chlorhexidine gluconate

Chlorhexidine gluconate has a broad spectrum of activity, although it is more effective against Gram-positive than Gram-negative bacteria. It binds to the *stratum corneum* and continues to destroy micro-organisms for at least six hours so that it remains effective for some time after application to the hands (residual activity/substantivity).[8] This is a major advantage in busy clinical areas in view of evidence that compliance with hand hygiene protocols reduces with increasing workload.[6] Substantivity is also useful when chlorhexidine is used as a surgical scrub, especially when the procedure is prolonged or surgical gloves become perforated. Chlorhexidine does not exert its bactericidal effects as rapidly as alcohol products, but after it has been used for several days, bacterial counts on the hands fall below their original level.[8]

Povidone-iodine

This is often used in operating departments because it is a particularly effective sporicide.[8] It also removes methicillin-resistant *Staphylococcus aureus* (MRSA) effectively from the fingertips.[10] However, its odour and colour are not appealing and allergy is common.

Triclosan

This is not much used in the UK, but it is useful for those who have developed hypersensitivity to the more commonly used products.

Alcohol-based products

These have gained popularity because they are cheap and can be applied quickly between different patients and clinical procedures. A range of alcohol-based products has become available: handrubs, gels and impregnated wipes. The active ingredients are: ethanol, isopropanol or n-propanol. Sometimes an alcohol-based product also incorporates another antiseptic, usually chlorhexidine or triclosan. When combined with chlorhexidine, the product gains substantivity, but otherwise the effectiveness of these products, although rapid, is short-lived. Alcohols have excellent bactericidal activity against most Gram-negative and Gram-positive bacteria, but have no effect on spores and some types of viruses, notably enteroviruses. Lacking detergent effect, they are not suitable for use in the presence of heavy contamination. The formulation must incorporate an emollient because alcohol de-fats the skin, leading to dryness, soreness and poor compliance.

How effective are alcohol-based products when used routinely by practitioners?

Compliance with hand disinfection protocols is notoriously poor. Early research demonstrated that health professionals washed hands less than half the times they should, whether they were observed directly[11–13] or using unobtrusive methods such as monitors attached to taps.[14] A number of reasons were advanced to explain poor compliance, including poor motivation,[15] dislike of the products (especially when they were perceived to be harsh to skin),[16] lack of access to suitable products[6] and lack of time.[17] Since the publication of these early studies, steps have been taken to improve compliance, infection control has received greater emphasis,[1,2] manufacturers have worked to increase the number of products available and there have been major attempts to improve formulations so that they are more acceptable. Nevertheless, compliance remains low and interventions intended to increase the frequency of HHD using any product do not provide sustained improvement for more than a few months.[4] The exception is Pittet's work in Switzerland:[7] continuing high levels of compliance were achieved by combining the use of alcohol-based products with intensive feedback on performance to staff, resulting in a 'continuous Hawthorne effect'. This is resource-intensive and very time-consuming.

Most studies evaluating compliance have focused on the frequency of HHD because this is the most straightforward aspect to document. However, the few authors who have employed more sophisticated methodologies have uncovered even more worrying deficiencies. Gould's study[6] reanalysed frequency data to establish the extent of compliance taking place after activities likely to leave hands heavily contaminated ('essential decontamination'). The results indicated that decontamination when hands were likely to be heavily contaminated occurred less than 50% of the time. The few studies that have examined technique of HHD also indicate that it is suboptimal. Taylor's early simulation studies[18] revealed that large surfaces of the hands received no contact with the 'disinfecting agent' (a coloured dye), so they were not really disinfected at all. Gould[6] developed a numerical scoring system to document excellence of technique that was suitable for use with larger numbers. Again, significant areas of the hands escaped contact. The mean score was 8.5 out of 12. Later modifications to the score show that the situation has not improved. The score was 6.29 out of 11 when hands were washed conventionally and 3.87 out of 7 when an alcohol handrub was used.[19]

Alcohol-based products are considered to offer the greatest advantages at times of heavy workload when staff move rapidly between different patients and different activities, without time to use a sink.[20] There is evidence that reliance is placed on alcohol-based products at these times. In Gould's study,[6] they were used more often as workload increased, but fewer essential HHDs were performed ($p<0.05$). In fact, HHD took place faster when alcohol-based products were used compared to traditional products and fewer hand surfaces received contact ($p<0.004$). These results indicate that when alcohol-based products are used at very busy times, HHD becomes more haphazard and hands are probably not physically clean after supposed decontamination. It has been suggested that alcohol-based products disinfect less effectively because they lack viscosity and 'slip through the fingers' with no time to exert bactericidal action[21] and that over-reliance on medicated products might promote a sense of false security.[22]

Today, excessive use of alcohol-based products could be promoting tokenistic use. Practitioners and managers are seduced into thinking that they are undertaking and promoting best practice when in fact practice is suboptimal and unsafe. The few studies that have addressed HHD technique indicate that particular care must be taken to ensure complete hand contact when alcohol-based products are used. Further research in this area is required to find ways of overcoming this problem.

Is there enough guidance on how alcohol-based products should be used to achieve safe practice?

The Infection Control Nurses' Association (ICNA)[23] emphasizes in its national guidelines that alcohols are not cleaning agents. When the use of alcohol-based products is appropriate, the ICNA advises practitioners to:

- Dispense the required amount (not stipulated) onto hands.
- Ensure that all hand surfaces are covered.
- Rub vigorously using the same technique recommended for hand washing until hands are dry.

More recent guidelines offered by the Hand Hygiene Liaison Group specifically in relation to alcohol-based products[24] advise health workers to:

- Pour 1–3 ml of alcohol handrub onto the cupped palm of one hand.
- Press the fingertips and nails of the other hand into the alcohol.
- Tip the remaining alcohol into the cupped palm of the other hand and repeat pressing fingertips into the alcohol.
- Quickly spread the remaining alcohol over the surfaces of the hands until they are dry.

This guidance does attempt to tackle the problem of ensuring full hand cover when using a product that will evaporate rapidly. However, the technique does not appear to have been widely tested in practice yet, and this is a drawback as the practitioner is expected to undertake a series of quite intricate activities very rapidly in the busy patient environment. Describing the technique, Jeanes[25] emphasizes that alcohol-based products should only be applied to physically clean hands. Overall, it appears that practical, evidence-based guidelines to ensure safe practice are lacking.

Is hygienic hand disinfection still the single most important infection control procedure in the NHS today?

HHD forms part of every other single clinical procedure and continues to be widely advocated in all literature and policy documents intended to tackle HCAI.[1,2]

Aesthetic desirability also dictates that hands should be thoroughly decontaminated between patients and between dirty and clean activities whether they involve the same or different patients. However, the condition of the clinical environment may also contribute to risks of HCAI in ways that have not yet been fully explored. Traditionally infection control experts[26,27] have considered that the inanimate environment has not contributed greatly to the risks of HCAI. This view is now changing[28] – possibly because the environment is now much more heavily contaminated than it used to be, especially in the UK. There is evidence that a wide range of clinical[29–31] and non-clinical[32–34] equipment is heavily contaminated. This begs the question 'What is the use of HHD?' when the health worker will immediately recontaminate their hands. When very heavy reliance is placed on alcohol-based products, the question becomes 'What is the use of a single episode of HHD without the added protection of regular traditional HHD using a longer-acting product?'

What other factors may be contributing to the relatively high rates of HCAI recorded in the UK?

In recent policy documents, unfavourable comparisons have been made between rates of HCAI in the UK compared with continental Europe.[1] The CleanYourHands Campaign has been designed to improve HHD compliance by introducing models of infection control that have been successful in other countries. However the UK, with its NHS, has a unique model of health service delivery that may reduce the success of schemes imported piecemeal from elsewhere. Idiosyncratic practices in the UK include the following:

Cleaning

Many other countries never abandoned environmental cleaning with surface disinfectants, but in the UK disinfectants ceased to be recommended for environmental cleaning in the 1980s.[35] There is now a turn in the tide of opinion concerning this issue.[36]

Lack of common sense concerning general cleaning and infection control

It appears that very complete instructions are required for some groups of health workers and that good supervision is essential to ensure compliance as intended.[34]

Shortage of specialist patient services

As a consequence of this, the same patient is likely to be moved between wards and Trusts, transferring their microbiological flora with them and acquiring additional pathogens on the way. This situation is exacerbated by the 4-hour target waiting period in the Accident and Emergency Department, because this encourages the use of shortstay wards and transfer to the first, often inappropriate, bed that becomes available, necessitating yet another move to a bed in the correct ward.

Centralizing critically ill patients in dedicated intensive care units

This practice increases opportunities for cross-infection between immunocompromised hosts. In some continental countries, each ward is equipped with its own small number of intensive care beds, reducing risks.

Retention of old hospital buildings that are not purpose built and lack adequate numbers of single rooms

Conflicts arise over the best use of rooms – for example when a highly infectious and a terminally ill patient both require the only single room available.

Blurred hospital-community boundary

In the UK, the same specialist nurse may deliver care to inpatients while maintaining a caseload of patients receiving all or most of their care at home. In this way, typical hospital pathogens are carried into the home and back to hospital. Premature discharge followed rapidly by readmission further exacerbates the problem.

Changes in the way in which equipment is used

More invasive procedures are being undertaken in outpatient clinics and day-surgery units. Pressure on the use of equipment has increased with high levels of patient throughput, and, as a result, local staff are in some cases being encouraged to decontaminate equipment rather than return it to the central sterilizing services department. Quality control is less stringent and errors of decontamination are more common, especially when staff have not received adequate training.[37]

Changing roles of health workers

NHS health workers are being subjected to pressure to expand their roles, sometimes assuming responsibility for tasks when they lack adequate training, especially in relation to infection risks. For example, senior nurses are performing many tasks that were once exclusively the province of doctors. More worryingly, healthcare assistants with minimal training are undertaking the major part of direct patient care. Infection control is now becoming part of mandatory annual updating for health workers, but recent research[38] shows that almost a third fail to access this training.

Conclusions

Despite rapid and excellent bactericidal activity, alcohol-based products are not always the best choice for HHD, because their effects are short-lived, they lack cleaning properties and, in order for them to be effective, there has to be a high level of user compliance – when compliance is known to be a major and intractable problem. In the UK, the wholesale use of alcohol-based products is being promoted prematurely. There is a lack of research concerning the effectiveness of these products under in-use conditions, lack of adequate guidance on safe practice and lack of consideration concerning the possible unintended consequences of replacing traditional products with alcohols. Controlling HCAI in UK hospitals is already more challenging than in many other European countries because of our unique, sometimes idiosyncratic, methods of health service delivery. Quick-fix solutions that apparently work effectively elsewhere may not work so well here, and indeed may introduce further problems.

References

1. Department of Health. *Winning Ways: Working together to reduce healthcare associated infection in England.* London: Stationary Office, 2003.
2. Patient Safety Alert t04. *Clean Hands Save Lives.* London: National Patient Safety Agency, 2004.
3. Storr J. The effectiveness of the national cleanyourhands campaign. *Nursing Times* 2005;**101**:50–51.
4. Naikoba S, Hayward A. The effectiveness of interventions aimed at increasing handwashing in healthcare workers – a systematic review. *J Hosp Infect* 2001;**47**:173–80.
5. Reybrouck G. The role of hands in the spread of nosocomial infections. *J Hosp Infect* 1983;**4**:103–11.
6. Gould DJ. Nurses' handwashing practice: results of a local study. *J Hosp Infect* 1994;**28**:15–30.
7. Pittet D, Hugonnet S, Harbath S, Mourouga P, Sauvan V, Touveneau S. Effectiveness of a hospital-wide programme to improve compliance with hand hygiene. *Lancet* 2000;**356**:1307–12.
8. Ehrenkrantz J. Bland soap handwash or hand antisepsis? The pressing need for clarity. *Infect Control Hosp Epidemiol* 1992;**13**:299–301.
9. McGinley KJ, Larson E, Leydon JJ. Composition and density of micro-flora in the subungal space of the hand. *Clin Microbiol* 1978;**26**:950–3.
10. Huang Y, Ole S, Kamiya A. Comparative effectiveness of hand-cleansing agents for removing methicillin resistant *Staphylococcus aureus* from experimentally contaminated fingertips. *Am Infect Control* 1994;**22**:224–7.
11. Albert R, Condie F. Handwashing patterns in medical intensive care units. *N Engl Med* 1981;**304**:1465–6.
12. Sedgwick, J. Handwashing in hospital wards. *Nurs Times* 1984;**80**:64–7.
13. Mayer JA, Dubbert PM, Miller M, Burkett PA, Chapman SW. Increasing handwashing in an ICU. *Infect Control* 1986;**7**:259–62.
14. Broughall JM, Marshman C, Jackson B. An automatic monitoring system for measuring handwashing frequency in hospital wards. *J Hosp Infect* 1984;**5**:447–53
15. Bartzokas CA, Slade PD. Motivation to comply with infection control procedures. *J Hosp Infect* 1991;**18**(Suppl. A):508–14.
16. Larson E, Killien M. Factors influencing handwashing behaviour of patient care personnel. *Am Infect Control* 1982;**10**:93–9.
17. Haley RW, Bregman DA. The role of understaffing and overcrowding in recurrent outbreaks of staphylococcal infections in a neonatal special care unit. *J Infect Dis* 1982;**145**:875–85.
18. Taylor LJ. An evaluation of handwashing techniques. Parts 1 and 2. *Nurs Times* 1978;**74**:54–5;108–9.
19. Chudleigh J, Fletcher M, Gould DJ. Infection control in neonatal intensive care units. *J Hosp Infect* 2005;**61**:123–9.
20. Voss A, Widmer AF. No time for handwashing? Handwashing versus alcoholic rub: can we afford 100% compliance? *Infect Control Hosp Epidemiol* 1997;**18**:203–8.
21. Ojajarvi J. Handwashing in Finland. *J Hosp Infect* 1991;**18**(Suppl B):35–40.
22. Banquero F, Patron C, Canon R et al. Laboratory and in vitro testing of skin antiseptics: a prediction for in vivo activity? *J Hosp Infect* 1991;**18**(Suppl 18):5–11.
23. *Guidelines for Hand Hygiene.* Infection Control Nurses' Association, 1998, 2001.
24. Hand Hygiene Liaison Group: www.handhygiene.co.uk

25. Jeanes A. Using alcohol handrubs. *Nurs Times* 2005;**101**:28–29.

26. Maki DG, Alvardo C, Hassemer C, Zilz MA. Relation of the inanimate environment to endemic nosocomial infection. *N Engl J Med* 1981;**307**:1562–66.

27. McGowan JE. Environmental factors in nosocomial infection – a selective focus. *Rev Infect Dis* 1981;**3**:760–9.

28. Dancer S. Mopping up hospital infection. *J Hosp Infect* 1999;**43**:85–100.

29. Block C, Baron O, Bogkowski B, Amit P, Rubenstein E. An in-use evaluation of the decontamination of polypropylene versus steel bedpans. *J Hosp Infect* 1990;**3**:173–8.

30. Gould DJ. The fall and rise of cleanliness in British health care and the nursing contribution. *J Res Nurs* 2005;**10**:496–510.

31. Man GS, Olapoju M, Chadwick MV et al. Bacterial contamination of ward-based computer terminals. *J Hosp Infect* 2002;**52**:314–18.

32. Avita-Aguero, M. Toys in a paediatric hospital: are they a bacterial source? *J Infect Control* 2004;**32**:287–90.

33. Stacey A, Burden P, Croton C, Jones E. Contamination of television sets by methicillin-resistant *Staphylococcus aureus* (MRSA). *J Hosp Infect* 1998;**39**:243–4.

34. Karas JA, Barker C, Hawkin L, Hoadley D. Turning a blind eye to vertical blinds in hospital wards. *J Hosp Infect* 2002;**81**:74–7.

35. Griffith CJ, Cooper RA, Gilmore J, Davies C, Lewis M. An evaluation of hospital cleaning regimes and standards. *J Hosp Infect* 2000;**45**:19–28.

35. Rutala WA, Weber DJ. Surface disinfection: should we do it? *J Hosp Infect* 2001;**48**(Suppl S):S64–8.

36. Ruddy M, Kibbler CC. Endoscopic decontamination: an audit and practical review. *J Hosp Infect* 2002;**50**:261–8.

37. Gould D, Drey N, Allan T, Berridge E. *Commitment to Nursing: The Contribution of Job Satisfaction, Family-Friendly Policies and Continuing Professional Development*. Report to the General Nursing Council for England and Wales, 2006.

Discussion

NEIL WIGGLESWORTH: There appears to be a prevailing view that increasing the frequency of hand washing somehow diminishes the importance of technique, i.e. that washing the hands many times, but not very well, is better than once with good technique. Is there a trade-off at some point?

DINAH GOULD: I think there may be a trade-off, but I do not know the point at which it occurs. This would be an interesting research project. It would seem to be common sense that if *all* of the surfaces of the hands are not decontaminated due to faulty technique then increasing frequency of hand washing is unlikely to rectify this. Observing people, it certainly seems that idiosyncrasies are ingrained: if someone misses a part of their hand when washing once, they miss it every time.

KEITH HOLLAND: If you could perfect hand washing technique universally, would the risk of HCAI caused by MRSA and other organisms fall to zero?

DINAH GOULD: No, because there is so much more than hand washing contributing to this problem. However, achieving one hundred percent compliance with good hand hygiene would certainly be half of the battle.

KEITH HOLLAND: Well, to rephrase the question, do you think that there is currently an overemphasis on hand hygiene to the extent of ignoring other important factors?

DINAH GOULD: That could be true. In today's hospitals, the broader environment is probably more important than people think. Furthermore, many years of observing staff demonstrate that aseptic techniques are frequently broached. Many healthcare workers have a rather limited understanding of aseptic technique.

MARTINA CUMMINS: Part of the problem is that medical students are no longer taught aseptic technique, whereas this used to be the first thing that they were taught.

DINAH GOULD: I agree – we need to catch people at the start of their medical training.

MARTINA CUMMINS: Can gloves be decontaminated?

DINAH GOULD: No, not if they are legally designated as single-use items.

DONALD MORRISON: Is any part of the hand more likely to carry and transmit pathogens?

DINAH GOULD: The fingertips are clearly more likely to be involved in intricate work, and other parts of the hand in ward work, such as lifting. As someone has already commented, the Ward Sister is the key member of staff for ensuring compliance with hand hygiene protocols.

DAVID GREEN: Senior medical staff are also important role models. In our Trust we have been looking at preparation for hand hygiene – by this, I mean the absence of long sleeves, no watches, jewellery, or charity bands. Despite reinforcing these messages, audits show that compliance remains low. We are asking our medical staff to take off jackets and roll up their sleeves when they come onto wards, and this does appear to be working.

Randomized clinical trials to support surgical hand antisepsis

Judith Tanner

Surgical hand antisepsis is carried out by all members of the operating team prior to undertaking invasive procedures. This is to reduce the potential for transferred pathogens resulting in surgical site infection. Despite being a well-known image of surgery, evidence to support hand antisepsis is limited. Most trials are conducted in laboratories and there have been few clinical trials. This contribution discusses the findings of a systematic review of surgical hand antisepsis.

Introduction

The inadvertent transfer of microorganisms to patients during surgery can result in postoperative surgical site infection (SSI). The incidence of SSI ranges from around 1% to 20%, depending on the nature of the surgical procedure.[1] There are numerous sources of SSI including transferred pathogens from members of the surgical team. In an attempt to reduce potential transfer, the surgical team undertake a number of preventative measures, including surgical hand antisepsis. Surgical hand antisepsis is intended to remove transient microorganisms and reduce or inhibit resident microorganisms.

There are three types of antiseptic solutions available for surgical hand antisepsis:

- aqueous scrubs
- alcohol rubs
- alcohol rubs with additional active ingredients

Aqueous scrubs

Aqueous scrubs are water-based solutions containing active agents or ingredients. The aqueous scrubs used most commonly contain chlorhexidine gluconate or povidone-iodine. Degerming the hands with an aqueous scrub requires performing a 'surgical scrub'. Scrubbing involves wetting the hands and forearms with water, applying an aqueous scrub using either palms or sponges, rinsing under running water then repeating this process.

Alcohol rubs

Alcohol rubs are alcohol-based solutions that are usually available in preparations of 60–90% strength. The three main alcohols used are ethanol, isopropanol and n-propanol and some rubs may contain a mixture of these. Degerming the hands with an alcohol rub requires performing a 'rub'. This involves a simple hand wash at the start of the day or whenever hands are visibly soiled to remove any dirt, then applying alcohol solution and allowing it to evaporate.

Alcohol rubs with additional active ingredients

These are alcohol-based solutions that contain additional active ingredients. Active ingredients include chlorhexidine gluconate, povidone-iodine, hexachlorophane, triclosan and chloroxylenol. The active ingredient is referred to as an additional agent as the alcohol itself is an active agent. Alcohol rubs with additional active ingredients combine the rapid kill of alcohol with the persistent chemical activity of aqueous scrubs. Degerming the hands using alcohol rubs with one or more additional active ingredients, requires the same process as an alcohol rub.

Recommended practices

Recommended practices for surgical hand antisepsis are published by numerous organizations including the Centers for Disease Control (USA), the Hospital Infection Society (UK), the Association for Professionals in Infection Control (USA), as well as perioperative nursing organizations such as the Association for Perioperative Practice (UK), the Association for Perioperative Nurses (USA) and the Australian College of Operating Room Nurses. However, these recommendations vary both between and within different countries. The variables debated include the relative effects of different antiseptic solutions, aqueous scrubs versus alcohol hand rubs and the duration of the procedure.

Despite the variations in recommended practices, surgical hand disinfection usually involves a simple prewash using soap, then the nails are cleaned with a brush or pick. The hands and forearms are covered with an antiseptic solution while applying friction (rubbing); this is then rinsed off under running water and the process is repeated. The first scrub of the day is referred to as the initial scrub and subsequent scrubs carried out during the remainder of the day are referred to as consecutive scrubs.

Surgical hand disinfection is costly in terms of both time and money. For example, rooms for the sole purpose of 'scrubbing up' are required adjacent to each operating theatre, with implications for the availability of antiseptic solutions and running water. Perhaps the most valuable resource consumed is personnel time, and the move towards evidence-based practice has necessitated a more robust demonstration of the clinical effectiveness of surgical hand antisepsis.

The first stage of the process of examining the clinical effectiveness of surgical hand antisepsis was to critically evaluate the existing evidence surrounding this practice. This called for a systematic review.

Methods – systematic review

Systematic reviews are recognized as providing the highest level of evidence.[2] They use explicit, systematic methods that limit bias and reduce chance effects, providing more reliable results from which conclusions can be drawn. Following an exhaustive search, studies are either included or excluded from the review, depending on their ability to meet predefined objectives and criteria. These objectives and criteria address the quality of trial characteristics, trial outcomes and design methods. Wherever possible, meta-analysis is carried out. Meta-analysis uses statistical methods to group together raw data from similar studies. This summary provides more precise estimates of the effects of healthcare rather than those from individual studies.

We wished to determine the relative effects of different antiseptic solutions, the effect of aqueous scrubs versus alcohol rubs and the optimum duration of hand antisepsis. The purpose of this review was to identify the clinical impact of surgical hand antisepsis; therefore, the primary outcome measure was surgical site infection in patients. However, the number of colony-forming units (CFUs) on the hands of the surgical team was identified as a secondary outcome. We were only interested in obtaining results from randomized controlled trials, as this design is universally recognized as providing the least opportunity for bias.[3]

The search strategy involved searching the following databases from 1966 to 2005: MEDLINE, CINAHL, the Cochrane Central Register of Controlled Trials and the ZETOC Database of Conference Abstracts. Around 200 potential articles were retrieved through the search strategy.

Three reviewers independently assessed the titles and abstracts of all retrieved articles, looking for potentially relevant trials. All potentially relevant trials were then independently assessed for inclusion in the review based on predetermined criteria, which included the quality of the trial characteristics, the trial outcomes and the trial design. The authors of two trials were contacted for further information relating to their trials. To date, one has responded.

A more detailed description of the methodology can be found elsewhere.[4]

Analysis

No trials were considered sufficiently similar to be included in a meta-analysis, therefore each study was considered separately. Where raw data were available from published trials, data was entered onto Cochrane RevMan 4.1 software and analysed using Cochrane Metaview to confirm the statistical analysis and interpretation of the trial author.

Findings – studies included

A total of seven clinical trials met the inclusion criteria and addressed the outcomes (SSIs and CFUs) referred to above. Two studies compared the relative effects of different antiseptic solutions (Tables 1–3). Five studies compared aqueous scrubs with alcohol rubs (Table 4). Three studies compared surgical scrubs of varying duration (Table 5). All of these seven trials are sufficiently different to preclude meta-analyses.

Discussion

Relative effects of different solutions

Chlorhexidine gluconate versus povidone-iodine (Table 1)
One trial[5] with four arms, compared chlorhexidine gluconate versus povidone-iodine for a 5-minute initial and 3-minute consecutive scrub and also a 3-minute initial and 30-second consecutive scrub. In the first comparison, chlorhexidine gluconate was more effective than povidone-iodine 2 hours after the initial scrub and 2 hours after the consecutive scrub while in the second comparison, chlorhexidine gluconate was more effective than povidone-iodine 2 hours after the consecutive scrub. This shows that, overall, chlorhexidine gluconate is more effective than povidone-iodine in reducing CFUs. It is not possible to comment on the sample sizes, as *a priori* sample calculations were not carried out.

TABLE 1 Chlorhexidine gluconate versus povidone-iodine: randomized controlled trial (RCT)

RCT	Intervention	Sample	Main results
Pereira et al 1990[5]	*Group 1*: 5-minute initial scrub and 3-minute consecutive scrub using chlorhexidine gluconate *Group 2*: 5-minute initial and 3-minute consecutive scrub using povidone-iodine *Group 3*: 3-minute initial and 30-second consecutive scrub using chlorhexidine gluconate *Group 4*: 3-minute initial and 30-second consecutive scrub using povidone-iodine	34 anaesthetic, recovery and ward staff rotating in a four-arm study.	*Group 1 vs Group 2*: chlorhexidine gluconate was more effective in reducing CFUs 2 hours after the initial scrub[a] and 2 hours after the consecutive scrub[a] *Group 3 vs Group 4*: chlorhexidine gluconate was more effective in reducing CFUs 2 hours after the consecutive scrub[a]

[a] Statistical significance.

Chlorhexidine gluconate versus povidone-iodine and triclosan (Table 2)

One trial[6] compared chlorhexidine gluconate versus povidone-iodine with triclosan for a 3-minute initial and a 2.5-minute consecutive scrub. No differences were found except for 2 hours after consecutive scrubs, which were taken after a week-long exposure to each product, when chlorhexidine gluconate was more effective than povidone-iodine and triclosan. This shows that, overall, chlorhexidine gluconate is

TABLE 2 Chlorhexidine gluconate versus povidone-iodine and triclosan: randomized controlled trial (RCT)

RCT	Intervention	Sample	Main result
Pereira et al 1997[6]	*Group 1*: 3-minute initial scrub and 2.5-minute consecutive scrub using chlorhexidine gluconate *Group 2*: 3-minute initial and 2.5-minute consecutive scrub using povidone-iodine and triclosan	23 operating room nurses rotating in a five-arm study	Chlorhexidine gluconate was more effective in reducing CFUs 2 hours after the consecutive scrub by day 5 of the trial[a]

[a]Statistical significance.

more effective than povidone-iodine and triclosan in reducing CFUs. It is not possible to comment on the sample size, as *a priori* sample calculations were not carried out.

Alcohol rub versus alcohol rub (Table 3)

One study[6] compared a 70% isopropanol-based alcohol with a 70% ethanol alcohol rub. There was no difference in the number of CFUs when either alcohol rub was used. Different preparations of 70% strength alcohol appear to be equally effective in reducing CFUs on hands. It is not possible to comment on the sample size, as *a priori* sample calculations were not carried out.

Aqueous scrubs versus alcohol rubs with additional active ingredients (Table 4)

Four trials[6–9] found that alcohol rubs with additional active ingredients are as effective as aqueous scrubs, and one trial[10] found an alcohol rub to be statistically more effective than scrubbing. The most influential trial[7] found that a 5-minute scrub with chlorhexidine gluconate or povidone-iodine was as effective as a 5-minute alcohol rub in reducing SSIs. This was a large, well-conducted trial. The remaining four trials[6,8–10] had comparatively small sample sizes and all measured CFUs rather than SSIs. One trial found that a 6-minute scrub was as effective as a 2-minute alcohol rub[8] and another that a 3-minute alcohol rub was more effective than a 3-minute scrub.[10] Another trial[6] found that a 3.5-minute consecutive scrub was as effective as a 30-second consecutive rub. The remaining trial[9] did not provide details of the duration of the scrub or the rub. The findings of these trials show that all scrubs of 3, 5 or 6 minutes (initial or consecutive) could be replaced by a 2-minute alcohol rub (this includes drying time), and consecutive scrubs of

TABLE 3 Alcohol rub versus alcohol rub: randomized controlled trial (RCT)

RCT	Intervention	Sample	Main result
Pereira et al 1997[6]	*Group 1*: 2-minute initial scrub using chlorhexidine gluconate followed by a 30-second application of isopropanol 70% and chlorhexidine 0.5%. Consecutive scrubs of 30-second application with isopropanol 70% and chlorhexidine 0.5% *Group 2*: 2-minute initial scrub using chlorhexidine gluconate followed by a 30-second application of ethanol 70% and chlorhexidine 0.5%. Consecutive scrubs of 30-second application with ethanol 70% and chlorhexidine	23 operating room nurses rotating in a five-arm study.	No difference in CFUs

TABLE 4 Aqueous scrubs versus alcohol rubs with additional active ingredients

RCT	Intervention	Sample	Main results
Herruzo Cabrera et al 2000[10]	*Group 1*: 3-minute scrub using chlorhexidine gluconate or povidone-iodine *Group 2*: 3-minute scrub using N duopropenide	154 members of the surgical team	N duopropenide was more effective in reducing CFUs post surgery[a]
Larson et al 2001[8]	*Group 1*: 6-minute scrub using chlorhexidine gluconate *Group 2*: 2-minute rub using 61% ethanol with 1% chlorhexidine gluconate	22 operating room nurses in a two-arm study.	Ethanol was more effective in reducing CFUs post surgery on day 5 only.[a] No differences in CFUs were found on days 1–26.
Parienti et al 2002[7]	*Group 1*: 5-minute scrub using either chlorhexidine gluconate or povidone-iodine *Group 2*: 5-minute rub using 75% R-propanol, isopropanol and mecetronium sulfate (Sterillium)	4387 patients in a two-arm study.	No statistical difference in SSIs
Pereira et al 1997[6]	*Group 1*: 5-minute initial and 3.5-minute consecutive scrub using chlorhexidine gluconate *Group 2*: 2-minute initial scrub with chlorhexidine gluconate, then 30-second application of 70% isopropanol and 0.5% chlorhexidine gluconate. Consecutive rubs with 30-second application of 70% isopropanol and 0.5% chlorhexidine gluconate *Group 3*: 2-minute initial scrub with chlorhexidine gluconate, then 30-second application of 70% ethanol and 0.5% chlorhexidine gluconate. Consecutive rubs with 30-second application of 70% ethanol and 0.5% chlorhexidine gluconate	23 operating room nurses rotating in a five-arm study	Both alcohol rubs were more effective in reducing CFUs immediately after initial disinfection[a] and 2 hours after consecutive rubs on day 5[a]
Pietsch 2001[9]	*Group 1*: scrub using chlorhexidine gluconate (duration unknown) *Group 2*: alcohol rub using 75% n-propanol, isopropanol and mecetronium sulfate (duration not known)	Sample size not known	Alcohol rub more effective in reducing CFUs immediately after disinfection.[a] No difference in CFUs after surgery

[a] Statistical significance.

3.5 minutes could be replaced by 30-second alcohol rubs. It should be noted that the regimes involving alcohol rubs incorporated a simple hand wash using soap at the start of each day.

Duration of the surgical scrub (Table 5)

Three trials comparing 5 minutes versus 3 minutes[5,6] and 3 minutes versus 2 minutes[11] found no differences in CFUs on staff hands. A 5-minute scrub was found to be as effective as a 3-minute scrub and a 3-minute scrub was as effective as a 2-minute scrub. However, a 30-second scrub resulted in significantly more CFUs than a 3-minute scrub.[5] None of these trials are considered to be methodologically high quality, and two trials[5,6] did not carry out *a priori* sample calculations. The findings of these trials show that all scrubs (initial and consecutive) could be reduced to 2 minutes.

TABLE 5 Surgical scrubs of varying duration

RCT	Intervention	Sample	Main results
Pereira et al 1990[5]	*Group 1*: 5-minute initial scrub and 3-minute consecutive scrub using chlorhexidine gluconate *Group 2*: 3-minute initial scrub and 30-second consecutive scrub using chlorhexidine gluconate *Group 3*: 5-minute initial scrub and 3-minute consecutive scrub using povidone-iodine *Group 4*: 3-minute initial scrub and 30-second consecutive scrub using povidone-iodine	34 anaesthetic, recovery and ward staff rotating in a four-arm study	*Group 1 vs Group 2*: 5- and 3-minute regime more effective in reducing CFUs 2 hours after the consecutive scrub[a] *Group 3 vs Group 4*: no differences in CFUs
Pereira et al 1997[6]	*Group 1*: 5-minute initial and 3.5-minute consecutive scrub using chlorhexidine gluconate *Group 2*: 3-minute initial and 2.5-minute consecutive scrub using chlorhexidine gluconate	23 operating room nurses rotating in a five-arm study	No difference in CFUs
Wheelock and Lookinland 1997[11]	*Group 1*: 3-minute scrub *Group 2*: 2-minute scrub. Participants could use either chlorhexidine gluconate 4%, chlorhexidine gluconate 2% or parachlorometaxylenol	25 operating room nurses in a two-arm crossover trial	No difference in CFUs after disinfection for 1 hour

[a] Statistical significance.

Quality of the studies included

Of the seven trials included in this review, only one study[7] stood out as being well designed and well reported. This was the only trial to measure SSIs in patients. In addition, this trial carried out *a priori* sample size calculations, it had sufficient randomization, testers were unaware of group allocation, and dropout rates and sample demographics were given. SSIs were measured using accepted definitions involving a 30-day patient follow-up.

The remaining six trials[5,6,8–11] measured CFUs, with one of these trials[10] using the fingertip touch test method rather than the standard glove juice test recommended for testing antiseptic products.[12] Only one of these trials[11] carried out *a priori* sample size calculations. In four of these studies,[5,6,8,11] the participants did not take part in actual surgery, instead continuing to wear a pair of sterile surgical gloves while they undertook circulating duties in the operating room. This may have had an impact on CFUs, as participating in stressful surgical procedures and working under hot operating lights might increase sweating. Finally, in two studies,[7,11] participants in the scrub groups were allowed to use different antiseptic solutions. Details of the randomization are poor in almost all of the trials.

Studies excluded

Twenty-eight randomized trials comparing different antiseptic preparations and alcohol rubs were conducted under laboratory conditions. Many of these studies addressed the requirements of the American Society for Testing and Materials E1115 test method for evaluation of surgical hand scrub formulations.[12] These involved participants having a 'washout period' lasting several days before commencing the intervention phase of the trial. During the washout period, their exposure to soap-related products was limited. In some studies, participants whose baseline bacterial hand counts were found to lie outside an accepted range were excluded from further participation. These trials did not meet the objective of the review, which sought randomized trials conducted in clinical practice, and were therefore excluded from the review. However, it might be interesting to compare the findings of the clinical studies included in this review with the findings of the laboratory studies.

Conclusions

An aqueous scrub containing chlorhexidine gluconate 4% is more effective than aqueous solutions of povidone-iodone and povidone-iodone plus triclosan in reducing CFUs on staff hands.

Alcohol rubs with additional active ingredients appear to be as effective as aqueous scrubs in reducing SSIs and CFUs. Therefore alcohol rubs with additional active ingredients are an acceptable alternative to initial or consecutive scrubs. Seventy percent strength preparations of alcohol rubs, using either isopropanol or ethanol, are equally effective. When using alcohol rubs, these should be preceded by a simple hand wash using soap at the start of each day.

Scrubbing for 5 minutes is as effective as scrubbing for 3 minutes, which is as effective as scrubbing for 2 minutes. Therefore initial and consecutive surgical scrubs using aqueous scrubs could be reduced to a 2-minute duration without increasing the number of CFUs on staff hands.

Recommendations for future research

Future trials of surgical hand disinfection should attempt to measure SSI in patients and use sample sizes based on *a priori* calculations.

Acknowledgement

This study was supported by the Association for Perioperative Practice and by Derby Hospitals NHS Foundation Trust.

References

1. Health Protection Agency. Surgical site infection surveillance in England. *CDR Weekly* 2004;**14**:1–5.
2. Muir Grey JA. *Evidence Based Health Care: How to Make Health Policy and Management Decisions.* Edinburgh: Churchill Livingstone, 1997.
3. Jadad A. *Randomised Controlled Trials.* London: BMJ Books, 1998.
4. Swarbrook S, Stuart J, Tanner J. Surgical scrubbing to reduce surgical site infection. *Cochrane Database Syst Revi*, 2003;(4).
5. Pereira LJ, Lee GM, Wade KJ. The effect of surgical hand washing routines on the microbial counts of operating room nurses. *Am J Infect Cont* 1990;**18**:354–64.
6. Pereira LJ, Lee GM, Wade KJ. An evaluation of five protocols for surgical hand washing in relation to skin condition and microbial counts. *J Hosp Infect* 1997;**36**:49–65.
7. Parienti JJ, Thibon P, Heller R, et al. Hand-rubbing with an aqueous alcoholic solution versus traditional surgical hand-scrubbing and 30-day surgical site infection rates. *JAMA* 2002;**288**:722–7.
8. Larson EL, Aiello AE, Heilman R, et al. Comparison of different regimens for surgical hand preparation. *AORN J* 2001;**73**:412–32.
9. Pietsch H. Hand antiseptics: rubs versus scrubs, alcoholic solutions versus alcoholic gels. *J Hosp Infect* 2001;**48**(Suppl, A):S33–6.
10. Herruzo Cabrera R, Vizcaino Alcaide MJ, Fernandez Acinero MJ. Usefulness of an alcoholic solution of N Duopropenide for the surgical antisepsis of the hands compared with hand washing with povidone-iodine and chlorhexidine. *J Surg Res* 2000;**94**:6–12.
11. Wheelock SM, Lookinland S. Effect of surgical hand scrub time on subsequent bacterial growth. *AORN J* 1997;**65**:1087–98.
12. American Society for Testing and Materials. *E1115 Test Method for Evaluation of Surgical Hand Scrub Formulations.* www.astm.org (accessed 2005).

Discussion

NEIL WIGGLESWORTH: It might be more appropriate to establish which is the best scrub and the best rub in each group, and then compare only these. Could I also ask why CFUs were chosen as an endpoint?

JUDITH TANNER: Most likely because they are easier to measure than SSIs.

GRAHAM AYLIFFE: It is also important to consider disinfection of the skin at the surgical site – surgical wound infection is a major problem. I suspect that hands are responsible for a relatively small proportion of SSIs.

KEITH HOLLAND: Just to be clear, is the hypothesis that some presurgical procedures undertaken by operating staff and on patients influence the outcome in terms of wound infections?

JUDITH TANNER: Yes – that some of these practices undertaken in the operating theatre impact on surgical site infections, including deep incisional infections.

KEITH HOLLAND: I think it would be incredibly difficult to set up such a trial, and it may not even be technically feasible. The state of the patient, whether they are immunocompromised, the type of surgery, and so many other factors could play a role.

JUDITH TANNER: Yes, but a certain type of surgery in a certain type of patients could be the experimental model used. Attempts could also be made to control for other variables.

KEITH HOLLAND: Microflora density on the hands and at the surgical site should also be measured in order to establish the correlation of CFUs and SSIs. It may be that the answer has nothing to do with density of microflora. I suspect that a very large and expensive trial would be necessary in order to arrive at a definitive answer.

JUDITH TANNER: I agree, but these constraints should not prevent us from trying to find clear answers.

ROBERT HILL: One problem of Cochrane Reviews is that so many studies have to be excluded, due to failure to control for confounding variables, not declaring sample sizes, or similar shortcomings.

The in-vitro and ex-vivo activity of antiseptics against MRSA

Zainab Al-Doori and Donald Morrison

Methicillin-resistant *Staphylococcus aureus* (MRSA) is a major cause of infections in hospitals, and its prevalence has increased dramatically over the last two decades. In 2004, MRSA accounted for 44% of *S. aureus* causing bacteraemia in the UK. In Scotland, the figure in the third quarter of 2004 was 40%. A dramatic rise in MRSA cases, from just under 600 to over 12,200, occurred in Scotland between 1995 and 2000. However, it is of note that between 2001 and 2005 there was no significant change in the numbers of episodes of MRSA bacteraemia reported in Scotland. As in the rest of the UK, the two epidemic MRSA clones (EMRSA-15 and EMRSA-16) are dominant in Scotland, accounting for 72% and 21% respectively of all MRSA referred to the Scottish MRSA Reference Laboratory. Three other international EMRSA clones have been reported, all of which have been isolated in Scottish hospitals over the last eight years.

Biocides, which include chemicals with antiseptic, disinfectant and preservative activity, are used in hospitals to prevent the spread of pathogens. Some agents, such as chlorhexidine and quaternary ammonium compounds (QACs), are used in all three capacities. Hand washing and hand rubbing, using various skin cleansing agents, are the most effective methods to prevent the spread of MRSA. However, with the widespread use of antiseptics both inside and outside the hospital environment, it is important that the continued effectiveness of various antiseptics against different MRSA clones be monitored. In addition, it is important that novel antiseptics or novel antiseptic formulations should be tested for effectiveness against the dominant MRSA clones in each country.

Biocide testing methods

As early as the 1950s, it became apparent to workers in the field of antibiotics, as distinct from biocide susceptibility testing, that there were many variables affecting these methods and that there was a need to standardize. This led in 1975 to the formation of the NCCLS, now designated CLSI (Clinical and Laboratory Standards Institute) in the USA. In Europe, there are at least six different national standards for antibiotic susceptibility testing. In contrast to the USA, European standards for testing the efficacy of biocides have only appeared in the last decade through CEN (European Committee for Standardization).

The effectiveness of various skin biocides/antiseptics can be determined using in-vitro assays, including MIC determination, suspension and 'carrier' tests, and in-vivo assays, including the forearm and hand wash tests on human volunteers. European Standard EN1040 (1997) is the first-line assessment (phase 1 test) of a biocide and simply asks whether the product has a bactericidal activity. The requirement of this standard is for at least a 5 log reduction in viable counts of the test organism. Phase 2/step 1 testing involves laboratory tests that 'closely simulates practical conditions'. In EN1276 (1997), this involves simulating 'clean' and 'dirty' conditions by the addition of 0.3 g/l or 3 g/l bovine albumin respectively to the test product. This standard requires that within 5 minutes, at least a 5 log reduction in viable counts of four referenced strains has been achieved. The referenced strains include *Pseudomonas aeruginosa, Escherichia coli, Staphylococcus aureus* and *Enterococcus hirae*. In addition, there is scope for the use of other strains if required. Phase 2/step 2 testing goes further and more closely simulates 'real-life' situations. For example, EN1499 (1997) involves measuring the effectiveness of biocides on the artificially contaminated hands of human volunteers (an in-vivo test). Unlike the previous standards mentioned above, the requirement of this standard is a comparative one: the log reduction of test organism must be statistically significantly larger than that obtained by a non-medicated hand wash product. As with all testing models, both in-vitro and in-vivo methods have limitations.

MIC testing of biocides

MIC (minimum inhibitory concentration) data provide a useful starting point for the investigation of antibacterial activity. We tested the MIC of triclosan, chlorhexidine gluconate and cetylpyridium chloride for a collection of 220 MRSA isolated between 1997 and 2000 in 30 Scottish hospitals. The isolates included a large number of clonal variants of the two dominant EMRSA clones – in Scotland EMRSA-15 (72 isolates) and EMRSA-16 (73 isolates) – together with 87 isolates of various other MRSA clones. The MIC method was based on NCCLS methodology using cation-adjusted Mueller-Hinton agar (Beckton Dickinson, UK) at a concentration range of 0.015–64 mg/l. The two epidemic clones, namely EMRSA-15 (MLST type 22 or ST22) and EMRSA-16 (ST36), had triclosan MIC_{90} of 0.06 mg/l and 0.03 mg/l respectively and chlorhexidine MIC_{90} of 2 mg/l for both clones (Table 1). Although the majority of other Scottish MRSA (SMRSA) clones had triclosan MIC_{90} of 0.06–0.125 mg/l, three clones, namely SMRSA-117, SMRSA-99 (ST247, also referred to as the Iberian clone) and SMRSA-105 (ST5, paediatric clone), had triclosan MIC_{90} of 4, 1 and 0.25 mg/l, respectively. The MIC_{90} for chlorhexidine of these three clones was 4, 4 and 2 mg/l, respectively. The MIC for the quaternary ammonium compound, cetylpyridium chloride were similar to those for chlorhexidine. The significance of the various MIC results, especially the elevated data, is difficult to assess. The data in this study correlate well with those found in an earlier study by Suller and Russel.[1] Similar chlorhexidine MICs were also reported by Cookson *et al*[2] who questioned whether these represented resistance or just an elevated MIC. Unlike antibiotic testing, there are no standardized definitions of resistance in MIC terms. It has been proposed[3] that for *P. aeruginosa,* a chlorhexidine MIC ≥50 mg/l should be regarded as indicating resistance. Russell[4] suggested that, by analogy with antibiotic resistance, isolates should be considered resistant to biocides when they are not inactivated by an in-use concentration or by a concentration that inactivates other strains of that organism. Decreased susceptibility to biocides has been variously termed reduced susceptibility, tolerance[4] or adaptation.[5]

MIC data, although useful, are limited to a measure of the extent to which an agent can prevent multiplication rather than bactericidal activity. In addition, biocidal activity may be affected by various factors, including the presence of organic material and pH, which cause partial or complete inactivation of the agent. In addition, Brill *et al*[6] showed that a basic factor such as the medium used to grow organisms before testing affected the in-vitro test result. Furthermore, care must be taken in relating the activity of the 'pure' chemical compound, as is often used in MIC assays, and the activity of the 'in use' biocide formulation, which often contains other constituents that can boost activity.

TABLE 1 The minimum inhibitory concentrations (MIC) against MRSA of three antiseptic agents.

Biocide	Type	Isolates tested	MIC range (µg/ml)	MIC_{50} (µg/ml)	MIC_{90} (µg/ml)
Triclosan	Bisphenol	220	0.015–4	0.03	0.06
Chlorhexidine	Biguanide	220	0.25–4	2	2
Cetylpyridium Chloride	Quaternary ammonium compound	220	0.5–8	2	4

In-vitro bactericidal testing of biocides

The two bactericidal assay models (suspension and carrier) will give a better representation of the biocide activity than MIC data. These two models, however, are different. One measures the effectiveness in a suspension while the other introduces the concept of a surface–biofilm interaction. When comparing the in-vitro suspension and glass carrier assay, Messager *et al*[7] found that activity according to the glass carrier assay was significantly lower for three of the four biocides tested. In addition, Maillard *et al*[8] found that in-vitro bactericidal assays overestimated the antibacterial efficacy of antiseptics when compared with the activity on an ex-vivo pig skin model. In bactericidal assays, it is crucial that the biocide neutralization step be effective, otherwise results will not be valid, as was shown by Kampf.[9] The bactericidal activity of two commonly used antiseptic preparations: 2% triclosan (Aquasept™) and 1% chlorhexidine as an aqueous preparation (Corsodyl™); plus tea tree oil (Thursday Plantation) and Aloe Vera (Topro™, Alliance Products), were all tested against EMRSA-15, EMRSA-16 and six other SMRSA clones using a quantitative suspension test method based on the European Standard EN1040. Serial dilutions were performed followed by the spot plate counting method of Isenberg. Aquasept and Corsodyl antiseptics gave a 5 log reduction of all eight clones tested after a 30-second contact time. The bactericidal activity of tea tree oil varied between different clones. However, a 5 log reduction was achieved for all clones after a 30-minute contact time. Topro aloe vera gave a 2 log reduction at a 30-second contact time; however, no further reduction was observed over a period of 6 hours. In another study in our laboratory six biocides were compared by suspension assay, including three formulations of chlorhexidine-based antiseptics (4% w/v chlorhexidine in a detergent formulation, Hibiscrub™; 4% w/v chlorhexidine, Hydrex™; 0.3% w/v chlorhexidine, Biocide-S™), 2% triclosan (Aquasept™), 7.5% w/v povidone-iodine (Betadine™) and a new investigational biocide formulation with a potentially long residual activity (Steri-X™). All products except Biocide-S gave a 5 log reduction of EMRSA-15 within a 1-minute contact time. Biocide-S, with the lower concentration of chlorhexidine, gave a less than 2 log reduction after a 5-minute contact time.

Ex-vivo skin model for testing of biocides

The in-vitro tests described earlier are useful to indicate the relative effectiveness of different antiseptics, but, unlike in-vivo tests, they will not necessarily reflect 'in-use' effectiveness on the skin. In-vivo assays, however, also have limitations, including difficulty in recruitment of volunteers, but especially, for ethical reasons, only non-pathogenic organisms and products whose toxicity and safety in human subjects is known, can be tested. In an attempt to overcome some of these problems ex-vivo 'skin carrier' models, using skin from animals, including pigs, dogs and cats[8,10] have been developed. Graham *et al*[11] used excised human skin from routine plastic surgery to measure virus survival rates. They compared virus survival on excised skin and metal disks and found that the half-life of the virus was four times greater on skin. This showed the significant advantage of an excised skin model over in-vitro carrier models. Maillard's group at the University of Wales in Cardiff take credit for realizing the potential of the ex-vivo human skin model for testing the efficacy of biocides.[7,12–14] They used fresh or frozen excised skin from breast or abdominal reduction surgery, and developed a simple Franz cell test apparatus. The ex-vivo model can be used to 'mimic' various in-vivo studies, including the standard forearm and hand wash assays, but can also be used to determine biocide residual activity. As with all models, the ex-vivo model also has limitations. The pH of ex-vivo skin (7.0–8.2) was higher than that of in-vivo skin (4.2–5.6), and differences were observed in lactate dehydrogenase LDH activity and oxygen consumption when these were used as markers of cell viability.[7]

In our laboratory, EMRSA-15 was tested against two antiseptics used in hospitals (Hydrex (4% w/v chlorhexidine gluconate) and Betadine (7.5% w/v povidone-iodine), a novel biocide (Steri-X) and two non-medicated soaps (Kimberly-Clark Hand Cleanser and Schulke & Mayr Sensiva™ wash lotion).

Fresh samples of skin were obtained with patients' informed consent after plastic surgery, mainly from breast and some from abdominal reduction. The skin samples were washed three times for 3 minutes each in sterile distilled water (to remove any residual antiseptics from the surgery) and cut to fit in the Franz diffusion cells (JB and DW Jones, Loughborough, UK) especially designed for the experiment with a donor compartment of 36 mm diameter (Figure 1). The receptor compartment was filled with Earle's balanced salt solution (EBSS, Sigma, Poole, UK).

The standard method mimicking the forearm test involved placing a 20 μl aliquot of culture inoculum containing about 6×10^8 CFU/ml on the *corneum stratum* of the skin, and the suspensions were allowed to dry for 3 minutes at room temperature. Then, 30 μl of biocide or non-medicated soap was placed over the bacterial suspension. A 'control skin', in which 30 μl of phosphate-buffered saline

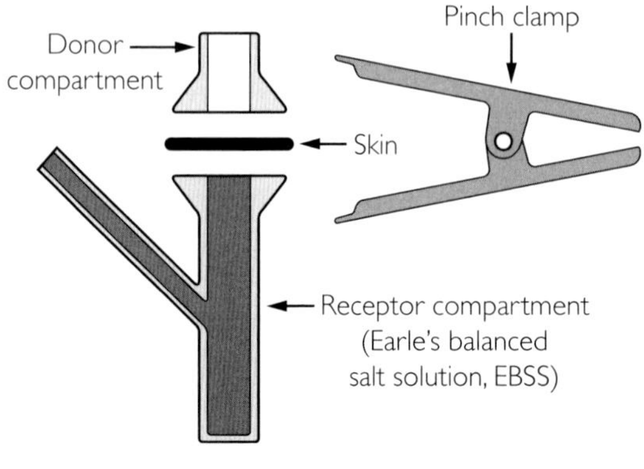

FIGURE 1 Franz cell

(PBS) rather than antiseptic/non-medicated soap was added, was included for every patient skin sample tested. After a 1-, 3- or 5-minute contact time, at room temperature, 450 μl of neutralizer was added and the surviving bacteria were resuspended (by pipetting up and down for 1 minute) and counted using the spot plate counting method. The hand wash mimic assay was similar, with the exception that following the 3-minute drying step, a volume of 480 μl of TSB was added to the skin and flushed by pipetting the TSB in and out of the pipette tip for 1 minute to give a 'prevalue'. A 40 μl volume of biocide or non-medicated soap was then placed on the skin and rubbed with a plastic loop for 3 minutes' contact time to give a 'postvalue'. To check for skin contamination, several samples of skin were tested by swabbing the skin sample prior to performing the ex-vivo assay. No bacteria were found on the skin.

In the forearm mimic test, Betadine and Steri-X gave over 1.5 log reduction and Hydrex an almost 2.5 log reduction (Figure 2). All three biocides were significantly more active than the Kimberly–Clark non-medicated soap at a 3-minute contact time. The difference between the activities of Hydrex, Betadine and Steri-X was not significant. When PBS alone (the control) was tested, this accounted for a less than 0.2 log reduction.

In the hand wash mimic test, Hydrex and Betadine gave 3 log and over 4 log reductions, respectively (Figure 3). They were both more active than the non-medicated Sensiva soap, although not significantly.

Preliminary work has been undertaken in our laboratory using the ex-vivo skin model to measure the residual activity of biocides. Biocide (60 μl) was placed on the *corneum stratum* of the skin and allowed to dry for 3 minutes at room temperature. The biocide on the skin was then repeatedly challenged with 20 μl of bacteria (6×10^6 CFU/ml), using a 3-minute contact time, at challenge times of 0, 2, 4 and 24 hours. Following the 3-minute contact time, 400 μl PBS was added, the surviving bacteria were resuspended (by pipetting up and down for 1 minute), added to the neutralizer solution and counted using the spot plate counting method. A 'control skin', in which 60 μl of PBS rather than biocide was added, was

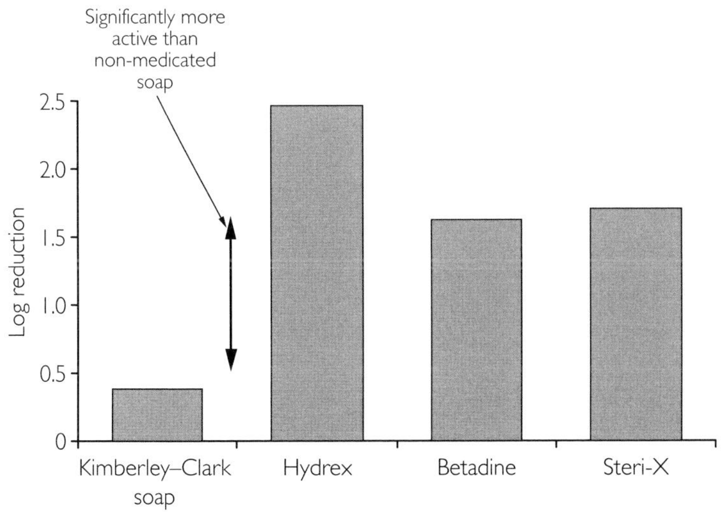

FIGURE 2 Ex-vivo forearm assay (3-minute contact time)

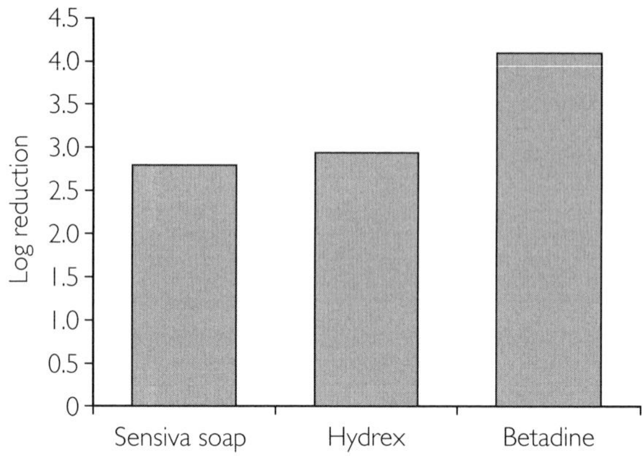

FIGURE 3 Ex-vivo hand wash assay (3-minute contact time)

included for comparison. Hydrex gave a 5 log reduction of EMRSA-15 at 0, 2 and 4 hours. At 24 hours, the log reduction obtained with Hydrex was only marginally better than with the PBS control. This result using an ex-vivo model confirmed the results of Ayliffe *et al*[15] who showed that chlorhexidine products had good residual activity over a 32-minute period.

Conclusions

It is important to measure the effectiveness of biocides used in the hospital environment. In-vitro studies give useful information about the relative activity of biocides, they can be used to study interaction with organic material, they are easy to perform and they allow large-scale testing to be undertaken. While in-vivo studies remain the 'gold standard' testing method, the ex-vivo model appears to be a highly suitable alternative with several advantages. In particular, it is easier to perform, it is cheaper, it allows testing under various conditions, pathogenic organisms and novel compounds can be tested, and ethical approval is easier to obtain.

References

1. Suller MTE, Russell AD. Antibiotic and biocide resistance in MRSA and VRE. *J Hosp Infect* 1999;**43**:281–91.
2. Cookson BD, Bolton MC, Platt JH. Chlorhexidine resistance in MRSA or just elevated MIC? An in vitro and in vivo assessment. *Antimicrob Agents Chemother* 1997;**35**:1997–2002.
3. Kampf G, Kramer A. Epidemiologic background of hand hygiene and evaluation of the most important agents for scrubs and rubs. *Clin Microbiol Rev* 2004;**17**:863–93.
4. Russell AD. Biocide use and antibiotic resistance: the relevance of laboratory findings to clinical and environmental situations. *Lancet Infect Dis* 2003;**3**:794–803.
5. Russell AD. Bacterial adaptation and resistance to antiseptics, disinfectants and preservatives is not a new phenomenon. *J Hosp Infect* 2004;**57**:97–104.
6. Brill F, Goroncy-Bermes P, Sand W. Influence of growth media on the sensitivity of *Staphylococcus aureus* and *Pseudomonas aeruginosa* to cationic biocides. *Int J Hyg Environ Health* 2006;**209**:89–95.
7. Messager S, Dettmear PW, Maillard JY. Determination of the antibacterial efficacy of several antiseptics tested on skin by an 'ex-vivo' test. *J Med Microbiol* 2001;**50**:284–92.

8. Maillard JY, Messager S, Veillon R. Antimicrobial efficacy of biocides tested on skin using an ex-vivo test. *J Hosp Infect* 1998;**40**:313–23.

9. Kampf G. Insufficient neutralization in testing a chlorhexidine-containing ethanol-based hand rub can result in a false positive efficacy assessment. *BMC Infect Dis* 2005;**5**:48.

10. Bush LW, Benson LM, White JH. Pig skin as test substrate for evaluating topical antimicrobial activity. *J Clin Microbiol* 1986;**24**:343–8.

11. Graham ML, Springthorpe VS, Sattar SA. Ex-vivo protocol for testing virus survival on human skin: experiments with herpesvirus 2. *Appl Environ Microbiol* 1996;**62**:4252–5.

12. Messager S, Goddard P, Dettmear PW, Maillard JY. Comparison of two in-vivo and two ex-vivo tests to assess the antibacterial activity of several antiseptics. *J Hosp Infect* 2004;**58**:115–21.

13. Messager S, Haan AC, Goddard PA, Dettmear PW, Maillard JY. Use of the 'ex-vivo' test to study long-term bacterial survival on human skin and their sensitivity to antisepsis. *J Appl Microbiol* 2004;**97**:1149–60.

14. Messager S, Hammer KA, Carson CF, Riley TV. Effectiveness of hand-cleansing formulations containing tea tree oil assessed ex-vivo on human skin and in-vivo with volunteers using European standard EN 1499. *J Hosp Infect* 2005;**59**:220–8.

15. Ayliffe GAJ, Babb JR, Davies JG, Lilly HA. Hand disinfection: a comparison of various agents in laboratory and ward studies. *J Hosp Infect* 1988;**11**:226–43.

Discussion

MATTHEW OLSEN: It would be useful to know if the pattern of resistance for the isolates was consistent relative to each agent tested.

ROBERT HILL: The question of whether there is resistance to antiseptics is interesting. There have been some reports of resistance to various antiseptics; however, inactivation by components of the culture medium should be considered when using MIC methods. Where MICs have been determined in-vitro, the culture media may interact with – and partially or totally inactivate – the antiseptic being tested, leading to a false indication of resistance.

KEITH HOLLAND: In the ex-vivo antiseptic assays, how are the bacteria removed from the skin sample in the Franz cell (i.e. taken off the diffusion-cell model)?

DONALD MORRISON: Once the sample has gone through the neutralization stage, a pipette is used to remove the bacteria and transfer them to the counting system.

KEITH HOLLAND: Many people use a detergent scrub to remove organisms from the surface of the skin. The use of this technique may lead to less variance in this model. Alternatively, once the sample has gone through the neutralization stage, a PTFE rod can be used to remove the bacteria and transfer them to the counting system. Some variability may also be due to the skin used in the model – some skin types have more sebaceous units, and consequently more microorganisms, than other types.

DONALD MORRISON: We flush our skin samples thoroughly because some have been pretreated as part of the work-up for the surgery during which the sample was collected.

MATTHEW OLSEN: Have you looked at variability due to age of the donor patient?

DONALD MORRISON: Ideally, we would like more information about the age and nationality of the patients from whom these samples were collected.

GRAHAM AYLIFFE: So there is no evidence that resistance is influencing antiseptic failures?

DONALD MORRISON: Our study with triclosan did not support the contention that widespread use will select for resistance in MRSA; however, our finding that some MRSA clones may have reduced susceptibility to triclosan highlights the need to be aware of such clones.

SHARON ANSON: The models described seem to be an excellent way of measuring transient organisms, but what about residuals?

DONALD MORRISON: We had not thought of that, but patients undergoing surgery will have had skin disinfection prior to theatre.

NEIL WIGGLESWORTH: Where did you get your MRSA strains from?

DONALD MORRISON: From our collection.

NEIL WIGGLESWORTH: You mentioned that you managed to induce increased MICs over time: is there any likelihood that in certain circumstances – for example if someone used a lot of triclosan for decolonization – that their 'local' strains may be potentially more resistant than 'generic' strains?

DONALD MORRISON: That is possible.

Development and testing strategies for antiseptics

Keith T Holland and Richard A Bojar

Antiseptics are widely used in the hospital and community environments, and their use should be a component of the strategy to reduce the risk of hospital-acquired infections. It is necessary to have methods based on robust models to test old and new antiseptics for their microbiogical efficacy, their capacity to drive resistance to themselves and other antimicrobial products, and their ability to cause skin irritancy. The object of this contribution is twofold: first, to highlight the diversity of testing that needs to be considered to develop and recommend products for risk reduction of transferring pathogens by skin contact in the hospital community; second, to suggest the direction for developing models that have good predictability for the efficacy of the antiseptic when used in the skin environment.

General considerations

The use of antiseptics in the hospital environment should be viewed as part of a strategy to control infections and cross-infections. Using antiseptics in isolation without due regard for other aspects of infection control will be unsuccessful and should be actively discouraged. Indeed, inappropriate use of antiseptic preparations in the hospital environment combined with widespread marketing to the general community, leading to excessive use external to hospitals, may compromise the long-term usefulness of some antiseptics.

Apart from the obvious microbiological issues associated with testing antiseptics, there are a number of practical aspects to be considered. For instance, the physical stability of the product will need to be tested, as widespread use in the healthcare environment will necessitate storage in less than ideal conditions. In addition, the effects on the normal functioning and condition of skin with frequent application should also be evaluated if compliance by hospital personnel, patients and visitors is to be maintained at the required level.[1] There are also issues with the persistence of antiseptic activity on the skin, with short duration antiseptics requiring frequent applications to be matched with staff activity. While products with persistent antimicrobial activity will reduce the frequency of application required and provide increased assurance, there may be consequences for skin irritancy, which may in turn adversely affect compliance. In addition, the general perception may persist that a product with residual activity can be used less frequently, thus having an adverse effect on compliance. There may also be implications for the selection of a resistant microflora, with suboptimal concentrations of the antimicrobial being present for longer due to infrequent reapplication.

The effectiveness of antiseptics against micro-organisms may be evaluated using a range of standard, validated testing procedures that are internationally recognized.[2] While these tests are useful for both consumer and manufacturer, they have limitations. The tests are generally pass/fail in nature. While this provides a clear message that a product that passes is an effective antimicrobial agent, the methods cannot dissect the subtleties of the mechanism of action. For instance, do ingredients of the product also accumulate in the environment, leading to selective pressure to encourage resistance in micro-organisms? Does persistence of ingredients on the skin encourage the transfer of resistance to pathogenic micro-organisms?

A coherent testing strategy must include monitoring of direct resistance to the product and evaluation of the possibility of linked resistance to other antimicrobial agents. Our society is educated to be aware of the need for good hygiene and cleanliness, which is a worthy goal in healthcare and in some household environments (e.g. the kitchen). However, over-zealous application of these principles to inappropriate situations, such as the domestic environment in general, can result in undesirable consequences of development of resistance in micro-organisms.

Generally, current antiseptics are effective against a wide range of micro-organisms, including the resident microflora of the skin.[3] At a conceptual level, the industry and healthcare professions need to discuss whether it is more desirable in future to attempt to develop antiseptics that have a minimal effect on the resident skin microflora so that there is little disturbance to the skin ecosystem with frequent use of the product. Likewise, more thorough testing regimes may detect products with an unacceptable propensity to encourage resistance.

Methods of testing

The microbiological activity of antiseptics may be evaluated using in-vitro and in-vivo model systems. Compared with in-vivo tests, in-vitro systems are usually considerably less expensive, are easier to control, with less variability, and are generally less technically complex. However, in-vitro models are less robust at predicting the activity of the product on human skin, particularly if only the pure active ingredient is tested in isolation. Consequently, in-vitro methods are best used as screening procedures prior to in-vivo testing.

The standard procedures for in-vitro microbiological testing of antiseptics follow the predictable methodology of traditional microbiology, using homogeneous suspensions of pure micro-organisms in a substantially aqueous environment. This is entirely different to the conditions on human skin, which is a physical surface with little free water, high concentrations of lipid, and communities of micro-organisms attached to the surface *stratum corneum* and in the pilosebaceous units at variable densities.[4,5] Therefore, it should be of no surprise that these methods have limited predictive capability compared with experiments carried out on human skin.

There is scope to improve the robustness of these in-vitro methods with the addition of components representative of skin, such as lipids and corneocytes However, while in-vivo methods must have greater predictive power, there are limitations to the scope of testing that can be carried out. For instance, it is not possible to test the effects on pathogenic micro-organisms in a controlled manner, as, for ethical reasons, these cannot be inoculated onto human skin. Such testing has to use subjects with natural contamination, who by definition may be patients undergoing treatment. A compromise approach is to use an indicator micro-organism that responds to the antiseptic in a similar way to the pathogen of interest but is itself non-pathogenic. Alternatively, the normal resident microflora of the skin can be manipulated to provide a suitable model system (e.g. elevating the density of *Staphylococcus epidermidis* under occlusion as a substitute for *S. aureus*).[6]

A compromise between in-vitro experimentation and in-vivo human volunteer studies is to use explant skin from humans. While ethical approval can be obtained for such procedures, in our experience the provision of tissue is at best erratic. In addition, the model system may have less predictive power compared with volunteer studies, and consequently the model is not widely used. Likewise, the use of animals or explant skin from animals is compromised by fundamental differences in the skin microflora and skin structure of humans and animals.

These problems can be overcome to a certain extent by using animals as hosts to accept transplanted human skin retaining its own microflora, but this is a sophisticated and technically demanding approach with all the combined ethical issues of animal use and the acquisition of the human skin. A further possibility, which is being pursued by the authors, is the development of a skin equivalent model colonized by bacteria. As an alternative mode, it has a number of advantages in that there are limited or no ethical issues to address, increased reproducibility, and no restrictions on the micro-organisms used and the level of destructive experimentation.

Standard tests

Microbiological efficacy can be evaluated using a wide range of testing procedures. The industry makes widespread use of standard methods with international (ISO, EN, ASTM) and local (BS) recognition. Individual test procedures can be used in conjunction with one another to evaluate different aspects of the antimicrobial process. For example in assessing the activity of hand rub products, bactericidal activity is initially demonstrated by in-vitro microbiology testing using prEN12054 (10^5 reduction in viable counts of *Escherichia coli, Psuedomonas aeruginosa, Enterococcos hirae* and *S. aureus* within 1 minute at 20°C), which is stipulated as a requirement for the in-vivo test of EN1500 (activity against *E. coli* on artificially contaminated fingertips of healthy volunteers) (BS EN 1500: 1997). Compliance with these two tests is recognized as a good indicator of product efficacy. However, it could be argued that the pivotal test of EN1500 merely demonstrates activity against faecal contamination with Gram-negative micro-organisms. The focus of infection control resources on Methicillin-resistant S. aureus (MRSA) in the healthcare environment has exposed some limitations in the EN1500 protocol, since this uses the Gram-negative *E. coli* as the indicator bacterium. *S. aureus* is Gram-positive, structurally different to *E. coli*, and may well have different sensitivities to that of *E. coli* to the products under test. It is possible, with minor modifications, to address some of the limitations, such as using *S. epidermidis* as an essentially non-pathogenic marker micro-organism for *S. aureus* and assessing activity against both *E. coli* and *S. epidermidis* without significant cost implications.

The industry's focus on passing tests such as EN1500 as part of the product development process has resulted in a situation where a product has to pass the test to make it to market, but this has resulted in EN1500 being devalued as a discriminator. Therefore, further modifications to the standard protocol, such as reducing the contact time from 30 seconds to 15 seconds, may act as a point of discrimination to identify products with enhanced antimicrobial activity. Indeed, it is also possible to argue that the reduced contact time of 15 seconds is more representative of 'in-use' conditions in healthcare environments, where it is often difficult to precisely perform the recommended hand decontamination procedure. However, we would suggest that full validation of any modifications should be undertaken in consultation with the wider infection control community.

Resistance development using chemostat cultures

Resistance to antimicrobial compounds in-vivo is primarily driven by the selective pressure imposed by exposure to the agent. In particular, sublethal concentrations are particularly effective at selecting variants within the microbial population with either higher levels of tolerance or genetic mutations conferring resistance. Ideally, antimicrobials should always be present in concentrations in excess of minimum bactericidal or fractional levels (MBC/MFC), or, at the very least, in excess of minimum inhibitory levels (MIC). However, while this is theoretically possible with systemic treatments, topical applications will always have a concentration gradient in the treatment area, and, at the periphery, concentrations will be suboptimal for microbial killing. Therefore, resistance to antimicrobials is always an issue with topical applications, and the mechanics of topical treatment mean that development of resistance is almost inevitable. While antibiotic compounds such as erythromycin rapidly select for resistance within the microbial population due to their specific mode of action, compounds such as benzoyl peroxide do not select for resistance as their mode of action is non-specific and consequently it is difficult for micro-organisms to develop resistance, even after prolonged exposure.[8]

Using indicator test strains with stability in prolonged culture and susceptibility to the antimicrobial agent, continuous cultures can be run using subinhibitory concentrations of the antimicrobial in the media feed. Viable cell counting over long incubation times, using non-selective growth medium (for total viable count) and media containing the antimicrobial at the minimum inhibitory concentration (MIC), 4x MIC and 16x MIC, will allow the kinetics of appearance and selection of resistant cells to be determined (Figure 1). This or similar methods should be considered for products used for reducing nasal carriage of *S. aureus*, for example.

However, these methods cannot predict the situation of environmental bacteria developing and/or acquiring resistance and transferring the resistance to pathogenic bacteria. Monitoring the environment for levels of antimicrobial accumulation and assessing the bacterial community for resistance should be considered.

Volar forearm occlusion model

Occlusion of volar forearm skin for 24–96 hours produces high population densities of the resident microflora. Volunteer studies may be undertaken under these conditions of high microbial load. This method is clinically more relevant and ethically more acceptable than alternative methods in which indicator micro-organisms are cultured in the laboratory and inoculated onto the skin prior to assessment. Under normal conditions, the microbial population of the volar forearm is relatively low ($< 3 \log_{10}$ CFU/cm^2) compared with the face, chest and back.

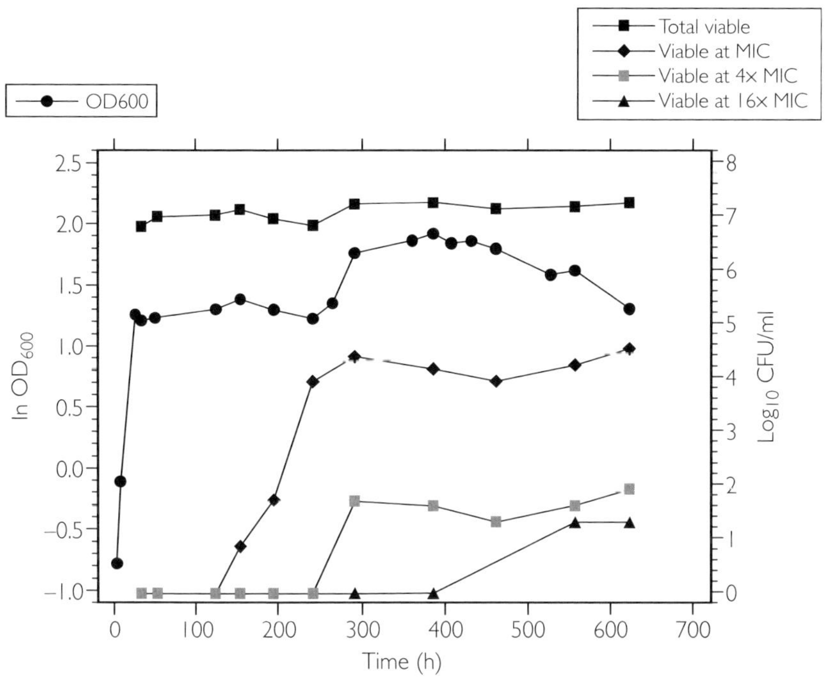

FIGURE 1 Growth and development of resistance by *Malassezia furfur* in the presence of an azole antibiotic

However, by occluding the skin with water-impermeable PVC tape, it is possible to produce a convenient model system for testing antimicrobial treatments. After a minimum of 24 hours occlusion, the resident microbial population typically increases by 2.0 $\log_{10}$ CFU/cm^2 and becomes dominated by *Staphylococcus* spp. (up to 99% of total population), a good indicator for *S. aureus*. The increased population density is maintained for at least 6 hours after removal of the occlusion, making the treated area ideal for testing the efficacy of antimicrobial preparations (Figure 2).

Colonized skin equivalent (CSE)

A living dermal/epidermal tissue culture model has been devised that can support colonization by micro-organisms that are resident on human skin and/or pathogenic species. The dermis can be based on a variety of matrices, such as fibrin or human decellularized dermis supporting human fibroblasts on which human keratinocytes are seeded and allowed to differentiate (Figure 3). The microorganisms are then applied to the *stratum corneum* surface and attach to this surface to initiate colonization (Figure 4). Antimicrobial agents can be applied to the CSE and the effect on the bacteria determined by a range of conventional microbiological techniques, including viable cell counting or measurement in real time of the luminescence from bacteria constructed with a lux reporter. In addition, the effect of the antimicrobial on the skin cells can be assessed using gene microarrays for human skin. The CSE model facilitates analysis for antimicrobial persistence and allows destructive assays as well as identifying products causing irritancy.[9]

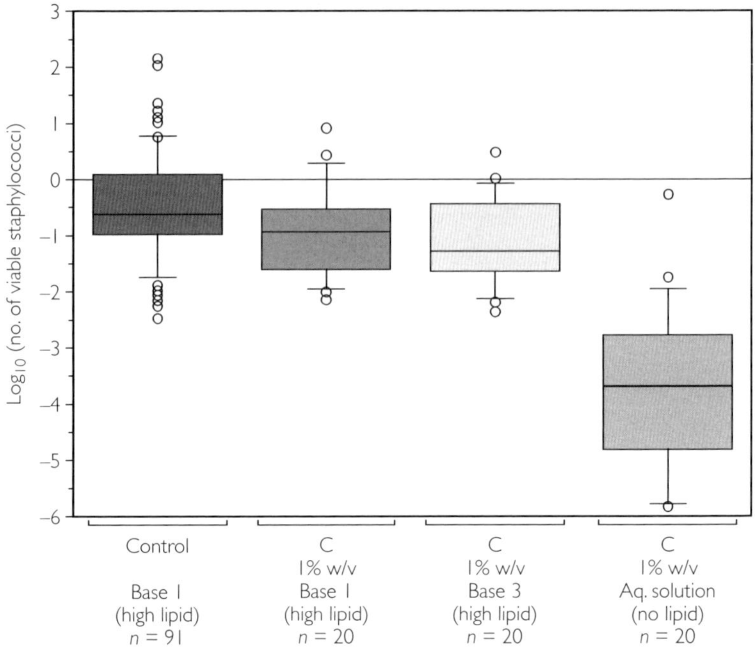

FIGURE 2 Number of viable *Staphylococcus* spp., compared with untreated control sites, isolated from the surface of volar forearm skin 6 hours after application of emollient base creams and an aqueous solution of compound (C) at 1% w/v. *n* is the number of replicates, with the data being presented as a box plot

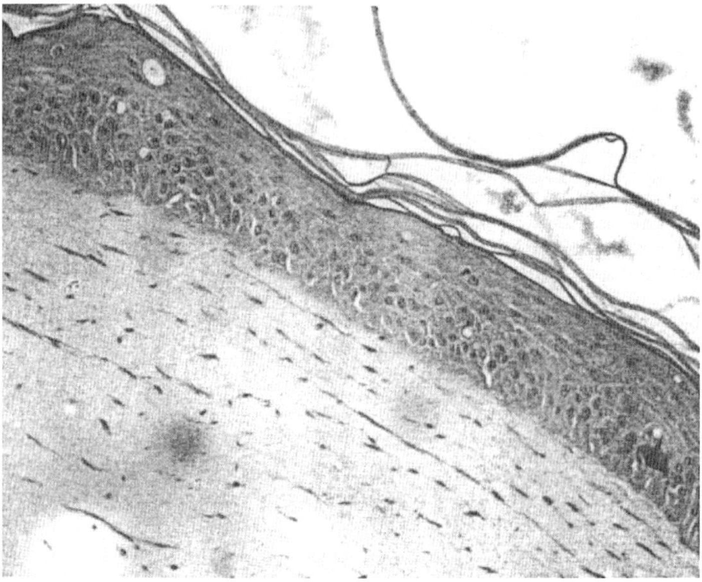

FIGURE 3 Stained section of a skin equivalent, showing a differentiated epidermis

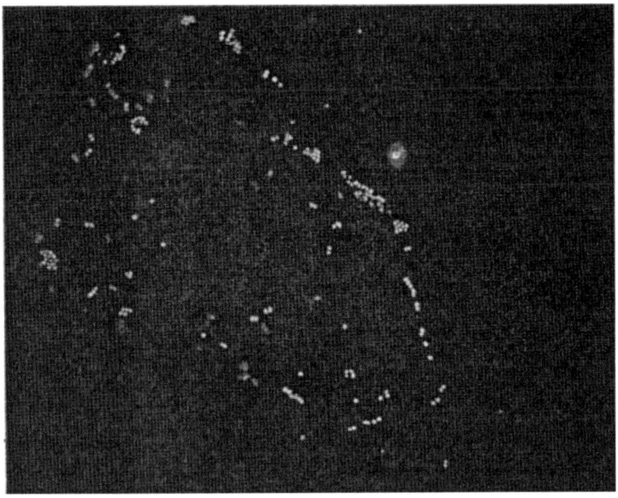

FIGURE 4 Live staphylococci labelled with a fluorescent probe on a corneocyte from a skin equivalent

Conclusions

Logic would dictate that tests of antiseptics in non-microbiological and microbiological ways, as well as rapid and low-cost in-vitro screening methods, are essential. Human models can be used to avoid animal testing procedures. The live skin equivalent model offers a valuable new technique, which should offer good predictability, with no ethical issues and employing a wide range of relevant pathogenic bacteria. Also, it can be used with destructive assay methods.

References

1. Lubbe J, Ruffieux C, van Melle G, Perrenoud D. Irritancy of the skin disinfectant n-propanol. *Contact Dermatitis* 2001;**45**:226–31.
2. Wendt C. Hand hygiene – comparison of international recommendations. *J Hosp Infect* 2001;**48**(Suppl. A):S23–8.
3. Adams D, Quayum M, Worthington T, Lambert P, Elliott T. Evaluation of a 2% chlorhexidine gluconate in 70% isopropyl alcohol skin disinfectant. *J Hosp Infect* 2005;**61**:287–90.
4. Leeming JP, Holland KT, Cunliffe WJ. The microbial ecology of pilosebaceous units isolated from human skin. *J Gen Microbiol* 1984;**130**:803–7.
5. Leyden JJ, McGinley KJ, Mills OH, Kligman AM. Age-related changes in the resident bacterial flora of the human face. *J Invest Dermatol* 1975;**65**:379–81.
6. Billhimer WL, Berge CA, Englehart JS, Rains GY, Keswick BH. A modified cup scrub method for assessing the antibacterial substantivity of personal cleansing products. *J Cosmet Sci* 2001;**52**:369–75.
7. Maillard JY. Bacterial target sites for biocide action. *J Appl Microbiol* 2002;**92**:16S–27S.
8. Ozolins M, Eady EA, Avery AJ, *et al*. Comparison of five antimicrobial regimens for treatment of mild to moderate inflammatory facial acne vulgaris in the community: randomised controlled trial. *Lancet* 2004;**364**:2188–95.
9. Rogers JV, McDougal JN. Improved method for in-vitro assessment of dermal toxicity for volatile organic chemicals. *Toxicol Lett* 2002;**135**:125–35.

Discussion

ROBERT HILL: Would the system you described be useful for looking at pharmacology?

KEITH HOLLAND: Yes. The Franz cell/explant system can certainly be used to look at perfusion of drugs, at persistence, at skin irritability (via interleukin -1a ELISA assay) and possibly at drug tissue distribution.

ROBERT HILL: What about small colony variants (SCVs)? They can intracellulize and have been associated with procoagulant activity in the vasculature and resumption of nasal carriage with the same strain.

KEITH HOLLAND: We found SCVs using this model – after 24 hours. It has made me wonder whether the skin equivalent model (SEM) can actually drive the selection of SCVs. However, this is not a predictable result – it does not happen in every SEM, so it may be more of a random mutation.

ANGELA KEARNS: Is there also strain variation?

KEITH HOLLAND: No. Incidentally, the strain that we are using incorporates a *lux* reporter.

Prevention of transmission of antibiotic-resistant pathogens by fingers: Role and determination of antiseptic half-life

Robert LR Hill

Hygienic hand disinfection (HHD) after each hand contact is essential to reduce healthcare-associated infection (HCAI). However, hand washing is universally irregular, and a schematic model has been formulated to analyse the potential effect of the half-life (*T½*) of HHD agents on non-compliant hygiene. The main factor determining *T½* is kinetic loss of applied agent from the fingertips. A contact transfer model taking account of kinetic loss has been used by volunteer subjects in an investigation of *T½* of an alcohol gel and an alcoholic chlorhexidine hand rub against antibiotic-sensitive strains of HCAI pathogens. Pig skin has been used in a variation of this model to investigate *T½* of test agents against antimicrobial-resistant pathogens. Preliminary results show that for antibiotic-sensitive *Staphylococcus aureus*, the *T½* of the chlorhexidine rub can exceed 24 hours and sustain over 2000 finger-to-surface contacts as a measure of kinetic loss. For resistant bacteria, including epidemic methicillin-resistant *S. aureus* (MRSA) and Multiresistant *Acinetobacter baumannii*, *T½* is about 15 minutes, but only a maximum of 100 finger-to-surface contacts are sustainable. The alcohol gel could not prevent transfer of antibiotic-resistant HCAI pathogens.

Introduction

Hand washing is emphasized as the single most important measure to prevent cross-transmission of micro-organisms and thus to prevent nosocomial infections.[1] Reybrouck[2] recognized that the purpose of HHD was to kill transient pathogenic bacteria contaminating hands, but, in addition, it should have residual activity to prevent further contamination until the next HHD. This is a very important observation, as in routine hospital practice, compliance with HHD is still unacceptably low – less than 50% in most studies published in the past 20 years.[3,4] This constant finding is worrying because, as recent modelling studies have shown, this level of compliance will not reduce the risk of transmission of multiresistant bacteria in hospital.[5] Attempts to improve compliance have included increasing the number of accessible sinks[6] and educating healthcare workers,[7,8] but none of these interventions has led to any marked and sustained improvement in compliance. As the ultimate solution, hand rubbing with an alcohol-based gel has been recommended and almost universally accepted as a substitute for handwashing.[9,10] Yet, in the UK at least, nosocomial infection has not abated, despite a significant tonnage of alcohol use. As little is known about the effectiveness of topical antiseptic agents for HHD in varying degrees of compliance, new thinking is required to tackle this universal problem.

This contribution will therefore consider a fundamental characteristic of all therapeutic agents (whether topical or systemic) that has been hitherto ignored in the application of HHD agents, namely that of antiseptic *T½*. Supported by preliminary investigations, this important parameter is to be considered in its widest context – that of its role in the use of HHD agents to combat HCAI.

Half-life of HHD agents

While little is known about the effectiveness of HHD agents, such as alcohol gels, in varying degrees of compliance, an important property of all therapeutic agents, that of half-life, has been ignored for HHD agents.

T½ is a novel concept for topical antimicrobial agents, requiring knowledge of the elimination rate constant, K_e. Evidence that *T½* exists, at least for some HHD agents, is exemplified by the residual activity of chlorhexidine on fingertips observed in the absence of finger-to-surface contacts.[11] Reybrouck[2] put forward the reasoning for using agents with residual activity, which can be readily equated with the concept and value of using agents with a significant *T½*, as expounded below.

As an established concept for systemic drugs, *T½* is the time it takes for the plasma concentration or the amount of drug in the body to be reduced by 50%.[12] Figure 1 shows the three main events associated with this: administration, circulation and elimination. *T½* exists because of elimination, and therefore determines the period for which active drug is available to the body and the time required for the concentration of that drug to fall by half.[13] This similarly applies to HHD agents, a dose being applied to the hands, circulated over them by rubbing action, followed by elimination, which (for a non-volatile agent), probably occurs by gradual elimination via the contact of other surfaces. There are few agents that are absorbed systemically, and these are not subject to consideration here. It is the thesis of this contribution that agents such as chlorhexidine, that are known to have sustained or residual activity on the skin are eliminated from fingertips via their contact with surfaces, to which an amount of agent is transferred and is lost from the original amount of agent applied.

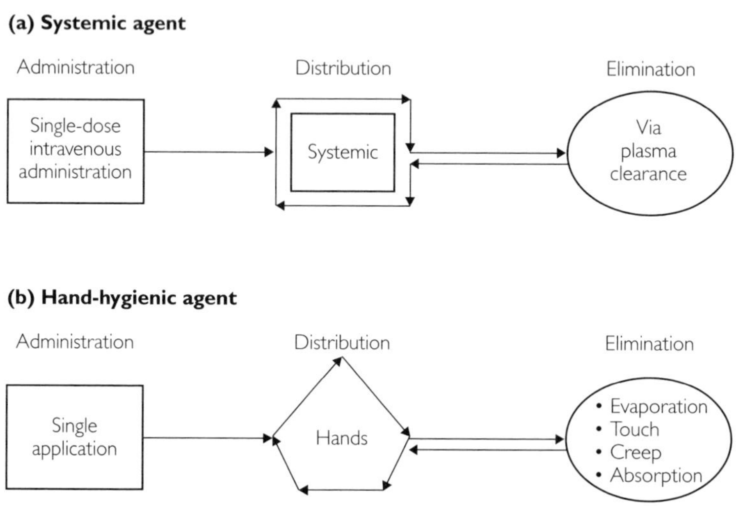

FIGURE 1 Pharmacology underpinning half-life

If we therefore consider HHD with antiseptic agents that are minimally absorbed from the skin, K_e can be calculated similarly to that for systemic drugs, with a modification of terms:

$$K_e = \frac{\ln C_1 - \ln C_2}{t}$$

where *C1* is the loading concentration on the fingertips and *C2* is the concentration after a set time *t*, which is defined by the maximum number of contacts that would reduce the concentration of the agent on fingertips to below that required to prevent acquisition and transfer of micro-organisms. Indeed, if *C2* is at the lowest viable concentration of HHD agent that would prevent cross-infection then $t = T½$. As one of the main losses of the applied agent is likely to be via finger-to-surface contact (ie. every contact transfers a proportion of the agent to the contacted surface), K_e and the number of hand-to-surface contacts are probably inextricably linked.

Theoretical determination of the significance of half-life

It is recognized that hand washing cannot prevent cross-infection, as absolute compliance is impossible.[9] It has been postulated that HHDA agents with a clinically significant half-life could help ameliorate the problem of missed hand washing oportunities.[14]

Schematic model

This schematic model is shown in Figure 2, and has been formulated because of two important observations:

1. It is probably not possible for healthcare workers to be cognisant of all contacts, that may involve the transmission of organisms.
2. As there will always be instances where handwashing is going to be missed, a general prophylactic measure is needed to 'cover the gaps'.

By randomly placing finger contacts and HHD occasions on the same time line, the period when fingers continue to be contaminated with bacteria can be determined. As the finger contacts and HHD occasions are unsynchronized, this represents non-compliance. The timing of the finger contacts and the *T½* of the HHD agent then determine the period of risk, i.e. when a contaminated finger can pass on pathogenic bacteria. The model assumes that (i) the first contact represents acquisition and following contacts transfer, until a HHD is applied; (ii) that the HHD agents completely eliminate bacteria from the fingers within their *T½*.

Figure 2 shows a 17-minute time line with four finger contacts and two HHD occasions. The risk periods for fingers passing on infective bacteria, when using HHD agents with theoretical *T½* values of 2 minutes compared with 15 minutes, are shown by the shaded bars. Despite the fact that the HHD agents each remove the contaminating bacteria, it is only the longer-acting agents that provide prophylaxis against further acquisition/transfer of pathogenic bacteria.

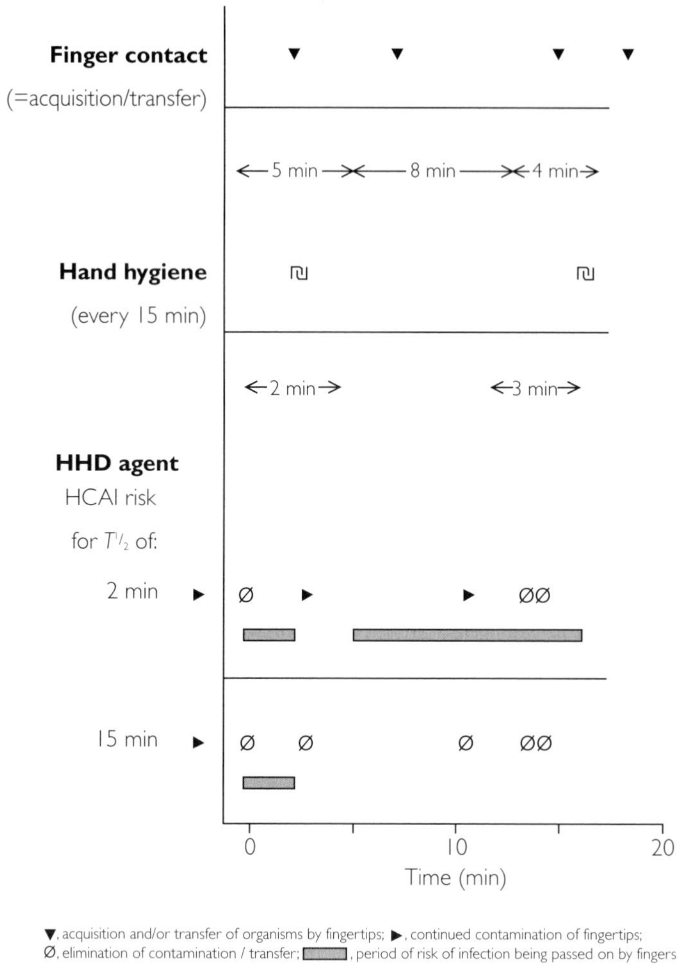

FIGURE 2 Model of the potential effect of the half-life ($T\frac{1}{2}$) of two hand hygienic disinfection (HHD) agents on the risk of healthcare-associated infection (HCAI)

Measuring half-life

Finger contact / transfer model

This is the basic test for determining the antimicrobial activity of an HHD agent on fingers, skin samples or artificial materials. The ability of HHD agents to prevent the transfer of organisms via fingers is also tested. Figure 3 shows diagrammatically the complete contact/transfer test procedure used with human volunteers: after application of an HHD agent to the hands of a volunteer, a finger is pressed onto an agar plate (Iso-sensitest, Oxoid, UK) seeded with a fixed density of colony-forming units (CFU), about 25 CFU/cm^2 of a non-pathogenic test organism, such as the Oxford staphylococcus (antibiotic-sensitive *S. aureus*, NCTC 6571). The finger is then pressed onto a sterile agar plate. After incubation (18 hours at 37°C for the bacteria described in the methods below),

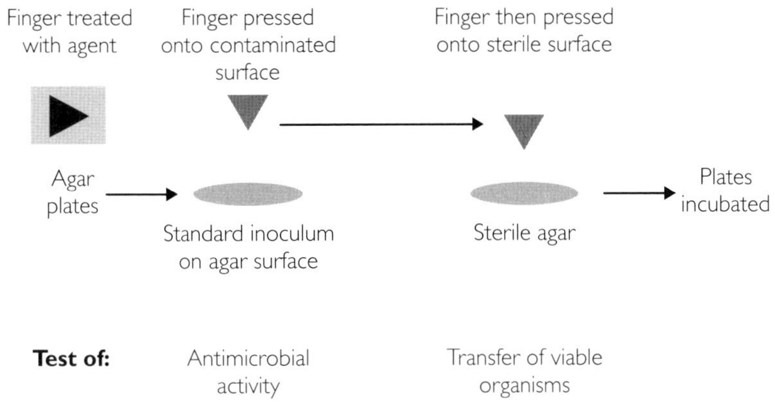

FIGURE 3 Finger contact/transfer laboratory model

the first plate will show a zone of activity around the fingerpad if the HHD agent is active; the second plate will only show colonies in the fingerpad if the HHD agent has not prevented acquisition and transfer of organisms from the first plate. Sterile water acts as the control agent. As it is unethical to inoculate the fingers of human volunteers with HCAI pathogens, the same method can be used with human or animal skin or artificial materials, to replace fingers. In this case, any pathogen can be used to seed the first agar plate.

In-vivo *experiments with human volunteers*

The time to extinction of antimicrobial activity of two HHD agents – an alcohol gel (62% alcohol, Go Jo Industries, UK) and a hand rub of 0.5% chlorhexidine in 70% alcohol (Regent Medical, UK) was determined on the fingers of healthy volunteers using the finger contact/transfer model as the basic measurement procedure. Ethical approval for these experiments was obtained from the King's Healthcare Trust Research Ethics Committee, London.

Hands were first prepared by hand washing with soap, followed by rinsing with water, then a rub with 70% isopropanol for 0.5 minutes, followed by rinsing with water and drying with a sterile towel. Two parameters were determined: first, the natural persistence of the agent on fingers held in air; secondly, the capacity of the HHD agent to withstand kinetic loss, simulated by finger-to-surface contacts using standard A4 printer paper as the contact surface. These are further described below; the indicator organism was the Oxford staphylococcus.

(i) Verification of the role of persistence

The hands and fingertips of volunteers were prepared as above. After application of the agent, fingertips were held in air at 20°C and pressed onto agars seeded as above, after set periods of time until extinction of activity to a maximum of 24 hours, as judged by the appearance of CFU in the fingerprint area. Sterile water was used as the control agent.

(ii) Verification of the role of kinetic loss (i.e. loss of agent from fingertips to contacted surfaces)

The agent was applied to the fingertips of volunteers after preparation as above. After the test agent had been applied, the fingertips were immediately pressed onto the surface of A4 paper (to effect standardized loss) for a varying number of times until extinction of antimicrobial activity, as judged by the number of CFU per fingertip imprint, after incubation. Sterile water was used as the control agent.

Antimicrobial-resistant HCAI pathogens

To negate the ethical problem of exposing human volunteers to highly transmissible multiply resistant hospital pathogens, the experiments in (i) and (ii) were replicated using 1 cm^2 of pig skin mounted on a 50 mm nail head. In order to remove bacterial contaminants and excess fatty deposits, the skin squares were washed in 70% alcohol. The Oxford staphylococcus was used as a control indicator organism; the test organisms were an epidemic MRSA (EMRSA-16), a multiresistant *Klebsiella pneumoniae* and a carbapenem-resistant *A. baumannii.*

Experimental results

Figures 4 and 5 show the natural persistence and resistance to active elimination of the two HHD agents. In both figures, the increase in CFU appearing in the fingertip print is commensurate with a decrease in the activity of the agent applied to the fingers. When the fingertips are held in air, there is no active elimination via finger-to-surface contact: only the natural persistence on fingertips is measured. While the activity of chlorhexidine in alcohol was undiminished after 60 minutes, the activity of the alcohol gel began to decrease after 1 minute (Figure 4). Chlorhexidine was also able to sustain 1000 finger-to-surface contacts without loss of activity against the Oxford staphylococcus compared with the alcohol gel, which sustained less than 5 contacts before CFU began to appear in the fingerprint area on both test agar plates (Figure 5). In further experiments, 2500–2750 finger-to-surface contacts were needed before the activity of chlorhexidine in alcohol began to decrease. The control agent (water) did not prevent acquisition and transfer of test organisms.

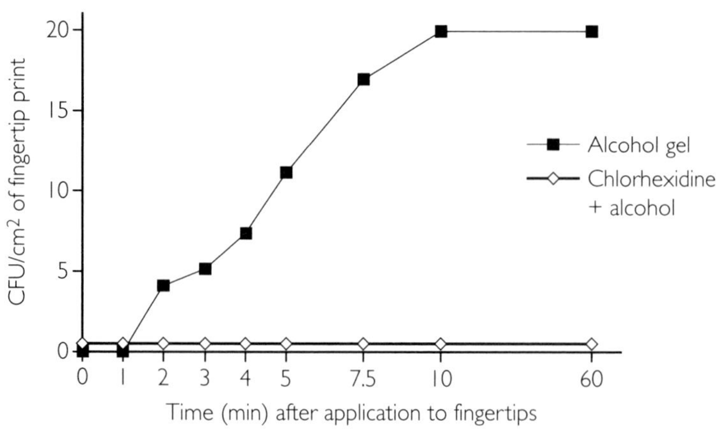

FIGURE 4 Activity of two agents against *Staphylococcus aureus* on fingertips held in air

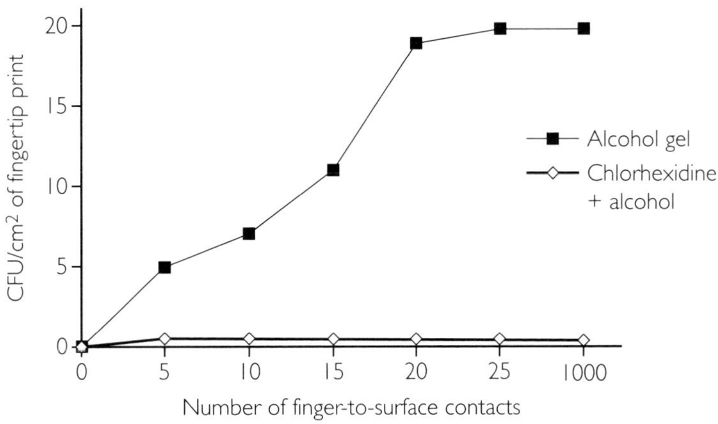

FIGURE 5 Activity of two agents against *Staphylococcus aureus* on fingertips after active elimination

On pig skin, the elimination life (*T*) associated with the Oxford staphylococcus was dramatically reduced (Table 1). *T*½ can be taken as half of this time. The most significant result was the reduction in the number of sustainable finger-to-surface contacts from 2500 to 500 (an 80% reduction). When antibiotic-resistant HCAI pathogens were tested on pig skin, values of *T* and hence *T*½, were further reduced by a similar order of magnitude. The alcohol gel had no activity against any organism on pig skin. While the *T*½ of chlorhexidine in alcohol on fingers or pig skin was a minimum of 15 minutes, the alcohol gel could only manage a *T*½ of less than 1 minute on fingers against the antibiotic-sensitive Oxford staphylococcus.

Discussion

Hand washing is the prescribed method for preventing cross-infection via hands, which accounts for at least 40% of HCAI.[15] Fingers have been shown to acquire organisms after brief contact with contaminated surfaces[16] and have been the focus of other models.[17,18] The concept of elimination of applied agents via contact with other surfaces is physically more difficult to measure with other areas of the hand, although it is acknowledged that palms and other areas may contribute to the transmission of infection. Thus measurements of antiseptic half-life have concentrated on fingertips.

The schematic model indicates clearly that the *T*½ of an HHD agent and the timing of hand contacts in relationship with HHD occasions are the important factors. Thus, for various frequencies or randomizations of hand/finger contacts that result in acquisition or transfer of pathogenic bacteria, the model can be used to determine the required *T*½ for an HHD agent. In practice, contaminating finger contacts could be at a higher frequency and the time between HHD occasions longer. By using data from various sources, the effect of different HHD agents can be predicted. For systemic agents, *T*½ is a derived parameter that changes as a function of both clearance and volume of distribution.[12] Similarly, in the absence of significant absorption, *T*½ for topical antiseptic agents is dependent on the ability of an agent to remain active on the skin and sustain kinetic loss, i.e. the amount of agent lost during finger-to-surface contacts. Thus, volatile agents such as ethanol or

TABLE 1 Elimination-life (*T*) and maximum number of sustainable finger-to-surface contacts for two HHD agents against antibiotic-resistant HCAI pathogens.

Test surface and organism	Chlorhexidine plus alcohol		Alcohol gel	
	Max no. of contacts	*T* (min)	Max no. of contacts	*T* (min)
Fingers				
Oxford staphylococcus	>2000	>1200	1	<1
Pig skin				
Oxford staphylococcus	500	>60	0	0
EMRSA-16[a]	250	60	0	0
Klebsiella pneumoniae[b]	100	30	0	0
Acinetobacter baumannii[c]	100	30	0	0

[a] Epidemic methicillin-resistant *Staphylococcus aureus*, type 16 (multiply resistant). [b] Colistin-sensitive only – ESBL producer. [c] Resistant to carbapenems.

propanol would not be expected to have a significant $T½$ even in the absence of kinetic loss.

The natural persistence of chlorhexidine in alcohol was shown to be high and is commensurate of previous findings of the persistence of chlorhexidine.[19] This is in complete contrast with the alcohol gel, which had very limited persistence. This would seem logical for a volatile agent applied to the skin, whose nominal temperature is 32°C. Similarly, alcohol sustained very few finger-to-surface contacts before loss of absolute activity occurred, which is commensurate with established findings of lack of residual activity.[19] This was in complete contrast to the remarkable capability of chlorhexidine to sustain active loss of agent from fingertips, which was in excess of 2000 finger-to-surface contacts. Again, this is commensurate with established findings of considerable residual activity.[19]

While the data from volunteers is able to prove the concept of $T½$ and show an extraordinary life for alcoholic chlorhexidine, the measurements from pig skin are quite alarming. On pig skin, the effective $T½$ was dramatically reduced, probably by partial inactivation of HHD agents by fatty substances associated with the pig skin surface. The number of contacts that chlorhexidine could sustain was brought down to 500 for the Oxford staphylococcus, which is a minimum reduction of 75%. Thus the elimination life T was tabulated rather than $T½$. On this basis, pig skin would not be the ideal choice for pursuing these type of experiments, despite being cleaned with alcohol to remove gross fatty material and bacterial contamination. Nevertheless, pig skin did show that, similarly, antibiotic-resistant organisms reduced T by some 75% compared with the antibiotic-sensitive control, although two of the most resistant and problematic bacteria currently in the UK were used in the experiments.

The $T½$ of an agent is therefore an indicator of dosing schedules, and, for a hand antiseptic, an increased $T½$ effectively lengthens the useful life of an application. Whilst little is known about the effectiveness of HHD agents in varying degrees of compliance, knowledge of the $T½$ of that antiseptic agent would help estimate the usefulness of an agent in ameliorating the problem of missed hand hygiene opportunities.

Acknowledgements

This work was carried out within the Department of Infection, King's College Hospital Campus, Guy's, King's and St Thomas' School of Medicine, London, UK.

References

1. Conly JM, Hill S, Ross J, Lertzman J, Louie TJ. Handwashing practices in an intensive care unit: the effects of an educational program and its relationship to infection rates. *Am J Infect Control* 1989;**17**:330–9.
2. Reybrouck G. Handwashing and hand disinfection. *J Hosp Infect* 1983;**8**:5–23.
3. Pittet D, Mourouga P, Perneger TV and the Members of the Infection Control Program. Compliance with handwashing in a teaching hospital. *Ann Intern Med* 1999;**130**:126–130.
4. Rotter, ML. Hand washing, hand disinfection and skin disinfection. In: Mayhall G (ed). *Hospital Epidemiology and Infection Control*, 2nd edn. Baltimore: Williams and Wilkins, 1999:691–709.
5. Austin DJ, Bonten MJM, Weinstein RA, Slaughter S, Anderson RM. Vancomycin-resistant enterococci in intensive-care hospital settings: transmission dynamics, persistence, and the impact of infection control programs. *Proc Natl Acad Sci USA* 1999;**96**:6908–13.
6. Preston GA, Larson EL, Stamm WE. The effect of private isolation rooms on patient care practices, colonization and infection in an intensive care unit. *Am J Med* 1981;**70**:641–5.
7. Simmons B, Bryant J, Neiman K, Spencer L, Arheart K. The role of handwashing in prevention of endemic intensive care unit infections. *Infect Control Hosp Epidemiol* 1990;**11**:589–94.
8. Bischoff WE, Reynolds TM, Sessler CN, Edmond MB, Wenzel RP. Handwashing compliance by health care workers: the impact of introducing an accessible, alcohol-based hand antiseptic. *Arch Intern Med* 2000;**160**:1017–21.
9. Boyce JM, Pittet D. Guidelines for hand hygiene in health-care settings: recommendations of the Healthcare Infection Control Practices Advisory Committee and the HICPAC/SHEA/APIC/IDSA Hand Hygiene Task Force. *Infect Control Hosp Epidemiol* 2002;**23**(Suppl):S3–40.
10. Boyce JM. Antiseptic technology: access, affordability, and acceptance. *Emerging Infect Dis* 2001;**7**:231–3.
11. Lowbury EJL, Lilly H, Bull JP. Disinfection of hands: removal of transient organisms. *BMJ* 1964;**ii**:230–3.
12. Wilkinson GR. Pharmacokinetics. In: Hardman JG, Limbird LE, Gilman AG (eds). *Goodman and Gilman's The Pharmacological Basis of Therapeutics*, 10th edn. New York: McGraw-Hill, 2001:3–29.
13. O'Grady F. Pharmacokinetics. In: *Antimicrobial Chemotherapy*. Ed, Greenwood D. Baillière's Concise Medical Textbooks, Baillière Tindall, London, 1983, pp.159–163.
14. Hill RLR. The half-life of handwashing agents on fingertips is potentially important for the amelioration of non-compliant hand hygiene. *Journal of Infection* 2003;**46**:P16–265.
15. Weist K, Pollege K, Schulz I, Ruden H, Gastmeier P. How many nosocomial infections are associated with cross-transmission? A prospective cohort study in a surgical intensive care unit. *Infect Control Hosp Epidemiol* 2002;**23**:127–32.
16. Scott E, Bloomfield SF. The survival and transfer of microbial contamination via cloths, hands and utensils. *J Appl Bacteriol* 1990;**68**:271–8.
17. Marples RR, Towers AG. A laboratory model for the investigation of contact transfer of micro-organisms. *J Hyg (Lond)* 1979;**82**:237–48.
18. Casewell MW, Law MM, Desai N. A laboratory model for testing agents for hygienic hand disinfection: handwashing and chlorhexidine for the removal of klebsiella. *J Hosp Infect* 1988;**12**:163–75.
19. Lowbury EJL, Lilly HA, Ayliffe GAJ. Preoperative disinfection of surgeon's hands: use of alcoholic solutions and effects of gloves on skin flora. *BMJ* 1974;**iv**:369–72.

Discussion

DONALD MORRISON: This is interesting work, but why not use explanted human skin rather than pig skin?

ROBERT HILL: Pig skin is readily available, more robust than explanted human skin and more readily fixable to a holding device, and it has been used in many experiments in place of human skin, including experiments with antiseptics. Mimicking or simulating normal human skin in experiments is a problem. The way round this in the work presented here was to control the experimental skin with that of human skin (volunteers' fingers) by means of an antibiotic-sensitive control organism – in this case, the Oxford staphylococcus.

KEITH HOLLAND: The results presented are interesting. Just to touch on non-microbiological issues, if manufacturers were to develop products with greater skin persistence, would these be more irritant to the skin?

MATTHEW OLSON: 'Skin-friendly' formulations are being developed and full irritancy tests are being conducted by dermatologists, using occlusive patch testing.

DAVID GREEN: Another potential drawback of agents with greater persistence may be that their use would lull users into a false sense of security and discourage compliance with hand washing. Perhaps we should develop persistent products but not broadcast the persistence?

DINAH GOLD: My experience of healthcare workers is that, above all, they want agents that are kind to their skin.

ROBERT HILL: Alcohol dehydrates the skin. Hand washing with soap may have similar effects. Hygienic hand disinfection formulations using water-based chemistry without detergents or alcohol could be usefully developed.

GRAHAM AYLIFFE: In the past, chlorhexidine cream was used in this fashion (rubbed onto the skin). We need to know more about the transmission of staphylococci from the hands and about the size of the inoculum needed to transfer infection.

EMRSA at the London Hospital: Comparing the early 1980s with today

Martina Cummins

Healthcare-associated infections (HCAI) or nosocomial infections are one of the most common complications affecting hospitalized patients.[1] For many years, it has been suggested that the hospital environment increases this risk to patients.[2,3] It has been reported that nine per cent of patients admitted to hospital in Britain acquire one or more infections, which adds an estimated £1 billion per annum to the cost of care.[4] However this was not a new situation, in the 1950s, there were national epidemics of hospital-acquired staphylococcal infections.[5] The introduction of methicillin as a treatment for *Staphylococcus aureus* infection in the 1960s became redundant over time as strains of methicillin-resistant *S. aureus* (MRSA) emerged. The next 10 years saw a dramatic rise in the prevalence of MRSA not only in England but also in other European countries such as Denmark, who reported a significant rise in the total number of *S. aureus* blood cultures attributed to MRSA.[6] By the early 1980s, the first outbreaks of epidemic MRSA (EMRSA) were reported throughout England. The outbreaks of this particular strain was identified by a specific antibiogram and associated with the ability to become endemic or cause outbreaks. One such outbreak at the Royal London Teaching Hospital, lasted over 4 years and at the time of publication had affected over 500 patients.[7]

The outbreak at the Royal London Hospital

Duckworth *et al*[6] discussed the five different phases of preventative measures that they used to try to bring the outbreak under control. These varied from cohort nursing in bays with the use of chlorhexidine nasal cream, body wash and shampoo, which had an initial impact, but was not sustained, as two months later cases were isolated on several wards.

It was noted that even with the use of side-room isolation on several wards, poor compliance or a lack of knowledge of isolation precautions resulted in a large increase in the incidence of EMRSA. This forced the radical decision to create an isolation ward.

The isolation ward, when combined with a new screening programme for both staff and patients in outbreak areas, plus the use of mupirocin nasal cream in the eradication protocol for positive individuals, formed the basis of the new control measures. Two years into the outbreak, it appeared that the infection control team finally had control of the problem, as the number of colonized or infected patients in the hospital and the bed occupancy of the isolation ward dramatically reduced.

Due to the reduction in the incidence of EMRSA cases and financial pressure, EMRSA-positive patients were cohort-nursed in bay areas of wards and the isolation ward was closed. However, a further outbreak ensued, necessitating the provision of a permanent isolation ward. The control measures were altered from chlorhexidine to 2% triclosan for washing patients in isolation and also encompassed an enhanced screening programme. This control strategy helped contain the outbreak, but EMRSA continues to be an organism that is not just a local problem but of increasing worldwide concern. A national prevalence survey conducted in 1997 reported that MRSA accounted for 15% of all hospital infections.[7] Deaths involving EMRSA subsequently doubled in 4 years and between 2002 and 2003. In 2005, the UK Office for National Statistics reported an astonishing increase of 20% in the number of MRSA deaths.

Formation of the St Bartholomew's and the London NHS Trust

Guidelines for the control of EMRSA in the UK were first issued in 1986, and were reviewed in 1990 and 1998, following changes in epidemiology, increasing prevalence of cases in hospitals and the community, major changes in the way in which healthcare is delivered, and the increased demands made on infection control teams.[6]

Following the merger of The Royal London Hospital and St Bartholomew's Hospital (Barts) (two large teaching hospitals) in 1994, common guidelines were agreed for screening and treatment to control MRSA across the Trust in line with the UK recommendations. We maintain a strict MRSA admission policy based on a search-and-destroy approach, ensuring that every reasonable effort is made to detect colonized and infected patients on admission. The policy dictates that only patients in high-risk groups are screened, which also include patients transferred from other hospitals, nursing and residential homes and those previously MRSA-positive.[8,9] Our policy also includes screening patients with a previous history of MRSA, as a study by Rodier and deWit[10] reported that these patients had a 62% chance of being colonized on readmission and recommended that they be identified, screened and isolated before admission to an open ward. The MRSA admission policy continues to include topical decolonization treatment, only now with chlorhexidine nasal cream (Naseptin™) three times a day and a daily skin wash and hair wash with Octenisan™ (a changeover from triclosan 2% used 12 months previously) until the screen is processed (approximately 5 days).

To accommodate the number of patients who may require isolation, a further 10-bedded isolation ward was opened on the Barts site. Admission to these beds continue to be controlled by the infection control team; however, we are now developing admission criteria for the wards to assist staff in identifying appropriate patients for these wards over night and weekends.

The use of preassessment clinics to screen all elective implant patients for MRSA carriage/colonization and treat all confirmed positives has contributed to the success of the orthopaedics in maintaining low rates of deep wound infections. Lidwell *et al*[11] state that this must not exceed 0.5%. The screening, in addition to ultraclean air in operating rooms and ring-fenced beds on the elective ward, has contributed to an overall reduction in infection rates. This is supported by Baint *et al.*[12]

One of the key principles in achieving adherence to infection control guidelines is to give staff a sense of responsibility for infection prevention and control. We have tried to achieve this by working with each directorate in the Trust and tackling issues that concern staff in their daily work. A good example of this is working with the renal and cardiac directorates to reduce line-related sepsis. The renal directorate in 2006 will have a nurse who will be responsible for line insertion and line care for all renal patients. By these means, we hope to achieve a 50% reduction in EMRSA bacteraemia by 2007.

Mandatory surveillance and reporting of *S. aureus* bloodstream infections for England and Wales started in April 2001. The Health Protection Agency Communicable Disease Surveillance Centre (London) has already reported outcomes through the Regional Epidemiologists, for NHS trusts for the period April 2001–September 2004. Until the 2004 data were published, Barts and the London had the lowest rate of MRSA bacteraemia per 1000 bed-days of any of the 10 specialist hospitals in London, despite the fact that a high percentage of the patients with MRSA colonization in St Bartholomew's and the London NHS Trust had acquired MRSA preadmission.

There is considerable diversity of control strategies across the North East London Sector, and this led to the agreement of minimum standards for MRSA control being agreed by infection control professionals and accepted by the North East London Sector Healthcare Acquired Infections Steering Group in December 2004. We have also developed an MRSA Action Plan to broaden ownership of the main issues at a local level.

What next?

We are not complacent in the products used for topical eradication (as mentioned previously we changed from 2% triclosan to Octenisan), and recognize the importance of having a good supply line and effective topical treatments. Due to an increase in resistance to mupirocin, we are currently reviewing products that may be an appropriate replacement for intranasal treatment. To reduce the laboratory time taken to identify MRSA from nasal swabs, we have completed a trial using a rapid (with results in about 2 hours) polymerase chain reaction (PCR) system. However, the technology that we used gave a high percentage of false positives. The poor sensitivity of this technology meant that it was not suitable for use in a hospital setting. We are currently trialling the Acolyte™ rapid testing method (with results in 5 hours), but further work is required if rapid testing is to be added to our screening policy, as it is only sensitive for nasal swabs.

By broadening ownership of infection control, it is hoped that we increase compliance with preventative measures. Research studies indicate generally poor compliance with infection control by healthcare professionals, which puts not only patients at risk, but also healthcare professionals.[13] The factors that influence this are access to facilities, busy caseloads where people feel they do not have the time to adopt appropriate practices, and a belief that what they have been asked to do is of little value to them and their colleagues. Becker *et al.*[14] suggest that lack of knowledge in relation to infection control appears to be a contributory factor to poor compliance. Kerr[15] found that successful infection control depends on adequate knowledge or correct application of knowledge, plus appropriate application of preventative measures to reduce the risk of cross-infection to patients. Prevention and control of infection activities are designed to limit the spread of infection and provide a safe environment for all patients, regardless of the healthcare setting.[16] Therefore, an education plan and basic infection control competencies for all clinical staff are included in the MRSA Action Plan – there is no longer room for complacency with regard to compliance with infection control measures.

References

1. Burke JP. Infection control: a problem for patient safety. *N Engl J Med* 2003;**348**:651–6.
2. Heseltine P. Has resistance spread to the community? *Clin Microbiol Infect Dis* 2000;**6**(Suppl 2):11–16.
3. Rothman KJ. Sleuthing in hospitals. *N Engl J Med* 1985;**313**:258–60
4. The National Audit. The management and control of hospital acquired infection in acute trusts in England. London: The National Audit, 2000.
5. Langmuir AD. The Epidemic Intelligence Service of the Center for Disease Control. *Publ Health Rep* 1980;**95**:470–7.
6. Jessen O, Rosendal K, Bulow P, Faber V, Eriksen KR. Changing staphylococci and staphylococcal infection. A ten year study of bacteria and cases of bacteraemia. *N Engl J Med* 1969;**281**:627–35.
7. Duckworth GJ, Lothian JLE, Williams JD. Methicillin-resistant *Staphylococcus aureus*: report of an outbreak in a London teaching hospital. *J Hosp Infect* 1988;**11**:1–15.
8. Cookson B. How to resist. *Health Serv J* 1987;**30** (Oct):9–11.
9. Office of National Statistics. *National Statistics*. London: HMSO, 2005. www.statistics.gov.uk
10. Duckworth G and the Combined Working Party of the Hospital Infection Society and the British Society for Antimicrobial Chemotherapy and Infection Control Nurses Association. Revised guidelines for the control of MRSA. *J Hosp Infect* 1998;**17**(3):7–35.
11. Duckworth G. Diagnosis and management of methicillin-resistant *Staphylococcus aureus* infection. *BMJ* 1993;**307**:1049–52.
12. Mulligan ME, Murray-Leisure KA, Ribner BS, *et al.* Methicillin-resistant *Staphylococcus aureus*: a consensus review of the microbiology, pathogeneses and epidemiology with implications for prevention and management. *Am J Med* 1993;**94**:313–28.
13. Rodier L, deWit D. MRSA colonisation rates of readmitted patients previously colonised with MRSA. *J Hosp Infect* 1996;**345**:86.
14. Lidwell OM, Lowbury EJ, Whyte W et al. Effect of ultra clean air in operating rooms on deep sepsis in the joint after total hip and knee replacement. *BMJ (Clin Res Ed)* 1982;**285**:10–14.
15. Baint LC, Teare EL, Williams WW, Tuite JD. Eradication of methicillin resistant *Staphylococcus aureus* by 'ring fencing' of elective orthopaedic beds. *BMJ* 2004;**329**:149–51.
16. Gershon RR, Vlahov D, Felknor SA, Vesley D, Johnson PC, Delcos GL, Murphy LR. Compliance with universal precautions among healthcare workers at three regional hospitals. *Am J Infect Cont* 1995;**23**:225–36.
17. Becker MH, Janz NK, Band J, Snyder MB, Gaynes RP. Non-compliance with Universal Precautions Policy: Why do physicians and nurses recap needles? *Am J Infect Cont.* 1990;**18**:232–9.
18. Kerr. J. Hand washing. *Nurs Standard* 1988;**12**(9–15 Sept):35–43.
19. Stucke VA. *Microbiology for Nurses: Application to Patient Care*, 7th edn. London: Baillière Tindall, 1993.

Discussion

GRAHAM AYLIFFE: This is impressive work, but I would hazard a guess that the cost of all these interventions is quite substantial.

MARTINA CUMMINS: It is very expensive, but overall we feel the expense is justified by the fact we are safeguarding our patients and reducing the risk of infection.

ROBERT HILL: If the NHS can find the funding to set up primary care trusts, why not find adequate funding to prevent EMRSA?

NEIL WIGGLESWORTH: When these protocols work, are they cost-saving in the long term, despite being expensive to run?

MARTINA CUMMINS: Well, we don't have many instances of MRSA-associated bacteraemia, however, mathematically modelling BLT data suggests that we have saved money on treatment and hospital stay. Although this was not our initial motivation – it is just part of our infection control programme.

SHARON ANSON: Some centres have performed cost-benefit analysis of MRSA screening versus the cost of dealing with outbreaks in terms of staff time, bad publicity, deaths, costs of treatment. In some cases, there have been overall cost savings.

DAVID GREEN: Have you considered doing slightly less screening, since only 1 in 16 swabs proves positive – why not refine the screening?

MARTINA CUMMINS: We have discussed this, but we have the laboratory support for our current screening frequency. It provides us with useful information, allows us to manage our isolation facilities and reduces the risk of cross infection, and it affords us the opportunity to undertake research on rapid testing. Also many other hospitals are now increasing their screening frequency.

NEIL WIGGLESWORTH: There have been published attempts to reduce screening by targeting patients on the basis of MRSA risk assessment – but this was not a success, because the authors could not find robust cut-off points for screening or not screening.

GRAHAM AYLIFFE: Some centres focus their screening on certain high-risk wards, such as intensive care units. It might help if we knew the accurate community incidence.

NEIL WIGGLESWORTH: A study currently in press shows a 22% MRSA nasal carriage prevalence in nursing home residents. The major risk factor was dependency.

DONALD MORRISON: Meta-analysis suggests a true community prevalence of about 2%.

GRAHAM AYLIFFE: I think Martina's presentation shows what we should do, if we could all afford it.

ROBERT HILL: The British Broadcasting Corporation produced a good documentary on the successful work on the control of epidemic MRSA at the London Hospital in the early 1980s, coupled with later failures. Entitled 'Intensive Scares – Killer Bug', 2003.

Closing remarks

Robert Hill

I would like to thank all of the contributors for their excellent presentations, which have covered a range of topics targeted at progressing the development of antiseptic agents for infection prevention and control of antibiotic-resistant pathogens. We have covered the new and challenging area of true community MRSA, clinical aspects of infection control and hand hygiene, plus some new and refreshing ideas and concepts concerning the clinically relevant analysis of antiseptic action. Undoubtedly, we need to take account of clinical processes and experience when developing laboratory and other models, to ensure good predictability for the efficacy of antiseptic agents when used in the clinical environment. There is also an urgent need for clinical studies that can fulfil Cochrane criteria.

This meeting has been a unique opportunity to bring areas of expertise together that might not otherwise be facilitated. On behalf of us all, I would therefore like to thank Regent Medical for their support and genuine interest in the subject matters discussed. In addition, I would like to extend our gratitude to MJM Communications for making the arrangements for the meeting itself and, together with Dr Ian Mason, for facilitating this publication. Last, but not least, I would like to thank Professor Graham Ayliffe for opening the meeting and for applying his longstanding expertise to our discussions.